staying Flexible

the full range of motion

staying Flexible

the full range of motion

TIME®
LIFE

by the Editors of Time-Life Books

CONSULTANTS FOR THIS BOOK

Charles B. Corbin, Ph.D., is Professor in the Department of Health and Physical Education at Arizona State University, Tempe. He is the author of several books, including *Concepts of Physical Fitness* and *Fitness for Life*, and has written numerous articles for scholarly journals. Dr. Corbin was honoured as a Prince Philip Lecturer by the British Physical Education Association and is a Fellow of the American Academy of Physical Education.

Risa Friedman holds a master's degree in dance education and is certified in health fitness by the American College of Sports Medicine, the International Dance Exercise Association and the Laban-Bartenieff Institute of Movement Studies. She has taught anatomy/kinesiology, movement analysis, therapeutic exercise, exercise physiology, and fitness and dance at New York University and the State University of New York, among other institutions. She is currently an exercise physiologist in private practice in San Diego, California, and is Program Director of the Fitness Specialist Certification Program at Marymount Manhattan College in New York City.

Judy L. Marriott is a Certified Movement Analyst with the Laban-Bartenieff Institute of Movement Studies and has worked as an exercise trainer since 1984. She is also a professional dancer and has performed with several companies nationally and internationally.

Marika E. Molnar is a physical therapist for the New York City Ballet. She is also a director at a Manhattan sports medicine centre and has lectured and written about the prevention and rehabilitation of dance injuries.

Myron Winick, M.D., is the R.R. Williams Professor of Nutrition, Professor of Pediatrics, Director of the Institute of Human Nutrition, and Director of the Center for Nutrition, Genetics and Human, Development at Columbia University College of Physicians and Surgeons. He has served on the Food and Nutrition Board of the National Academy of Sciences and is the author of many books, including *Your Personalized Health Profile*.

This edition published in 2005
by the Caxton Publishing Group
20 Bloomsbury Street, London WC1B 3JH

Under license from Time-Life Books BV.

Cover Design: Open Door Limited, Rutland UK

Editor: Charles L. Mee Jr..
Senior Editor: Thomas Dickey
Managing Editor: Susan Bronson
Senior Writer: William Dunnett
Associate Editors: Nona Cleland, Carl Lowe
Contributing Editor: Paul Perry
Art Director: Robin Schiff
Designer: Deborah Ragasto
Photographer: Steven Mays
Photo Stylist: Nola Lopez

Recipe Editor: Bonnie J. Slotnick
Contributing Editor, Food: Marya Dalrymple
Test Kitchen Director: Anne Disrude
Consulting Editor, Food: Sally Schneider
Nutritional Analyst: Hill Nutrition Associates
Chief of Research: Carney Mimms III
Assistant Editor: Jacqueline Dillon

Title: Staying Flexible

ISBN: 1 84447 165 9

This book is not intended as a substitute for the advice of a physician. Readers who have or suspect they may have specific medical problems, especially those involving muscles and joints, should consult a physician before beginning any programme of strenuous physical exercise.

CONTENTS

CHAPTER ONE

Flexibility

*Lengthening muscles
with the right stretches for
greater agility, better posture and
insurance against injury*

Physical fitness is more than just endurance or muscular strength. It is a complex latticework of many interrelated factors, each important in its own way. One of these factors is flexibility. Perhaps the most neglected aspect of many fitness programmes, flexibility training is being increasingly recognized as crucial for complementing muscular strength, building efficiency and co-ordination, and preventing injuries.

What is flexibility?
Flexibility is the mobility or range of motion in a joint. This range of motion is determined by the natural structure of the joint itself and by the direction in which it bends. Ball-and-socket joints, such as those in your hips and shoulders, afford greater range of motion than the hinge joints in your knees and elbows, the condyloid joints in your wrists, the pivot joints in your spinal column or the gliding joints in the metatarsals of your feet.

A joint is flexible when the muscles and connective tissues around it

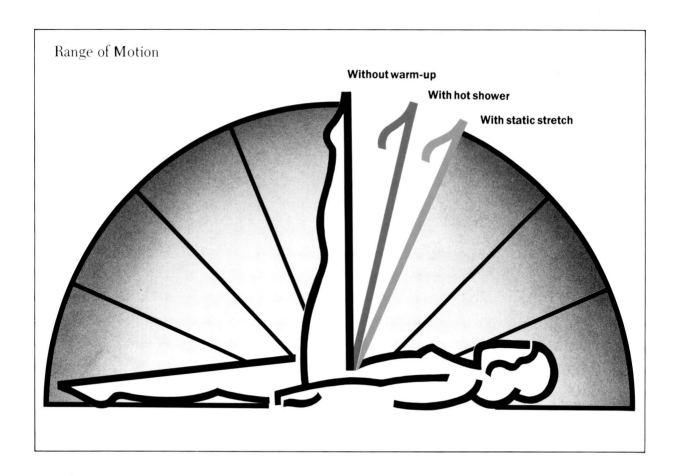

Without warm-up

With hot shower

With static stretch

A five-minute shower under hot water (43-45°C) will increase the flexibility of your hip joint so that it can move 5 per cent farther than it can when you are not warmed up. Static stretching can increase your range of motion by another 2 to 4 per cent.

do not restrict its natural range of motion. You should, for example, be able to extend your arm straight out at a 90-degree angle from your body and then flex your elbow joint enough to rest your hand comfortably on your shoulder. A flexible elbow joint allows full extension and flexion of your arm.

What limits flexibility?

When a joint moves, resistance from soft tissue is the major obstacle to its full natural range of movement. Researchers have determined that skin provides 2 per cent of that resistance, tendons and ligaments 10 per cent, and muscle tissue and its connecting fascia 41 per cent. The remaining resistance is in the joint capsule itself. Since the joint capsule, tendons and ligaments are composed of collagen, a non-elastic connective tissue, the length of muscles — which are both elastic and extensible — is usually the determining factor in the joint's range of motion. A "short" muscle limits range of motion; a "long" muscle allows a full, natural range of motion.

Are some people naturally more flexible than others?

Yes, but there is no ideal or standard for flexibility. The only standards available are based on norms that indicate how hundreds of individuals of both sexes and various age groups have performed. Generally speaking, tests have shown that children are more flexible than adults and that women are more flexible than men. Two studies, for instance, tested the flexibility of 510 males aged 18 to 71 and 407 females aged 18 to 74. These studies found that, for the average man tested, flexibility is greatest for most muscle groups and joints between the ages of 23 and 24; for women, it is greatest between the ages of 25 and 29.

Another study measured the flexibility of 300 randomly selected girls between the ages of six and 18. In most of the 12 flexibility measurements the researchers took, the girls' flexibility increased from the age of six to the age of 12 and then showed a decline. But the results were inconsistent: in terms of shoulder, knee and hip flexibility, there was a decrease between the ages of six and 18; yet 18-year-olds were more flexible in their trunk and wrist muscles and had better flexibility in the muscles along the outside of their thighs than the younger girls.

Is there a simple way to test flexibility?

For a long time, it was thought that flexibility was a general characteristic of the body: you were either flexible or you were not. However, researchers have now determined that flexibility is not equally apparent in all joints of the body. Just as there is a great range of flexibility among individuals in the same age and sex group, studies show that flexibility can even change drastically from one muscle group to another. In the study of 300 girls cited above, for instance, no girl was above or below average in all measurements of flexibility. You can have tight hamstrings and supple shoulder muscles, or tight hip flexors but flexible trunk muscles. You can even have bilateral differences in flexibility — your right quadriceps, for example, can be less flexible than your left quadriceps.

Flexibility in a joint also changes according to the direction in which the joint moves. You can be quite flexible when you bend your arm in one direction, for example, but less flexible when you use different muscles to rotate your arm in another direction. Also, the relation of one joint to another may influence the range of motion in one or both joints. For instance, if you are like most people, you can easily flex your fingers and tuck them into the palm of your hand so long as your wrist is extended. But if you flex your wrist, you will significantly reduce the range of motion in your finger joints, and you may not be able to tuck your fingers into your palm.

Clearly, flexibility is highly specific, making it difficult to provide an overall measurement without testing virtually every joint in the body. But you can get a general idea of your level of flexibility by taking several key measurements. The tests on pages 18-19 will help you define your own level of flexibility.

Why is staying flexible important?

For the athletic person, most experts believe that good flexibility

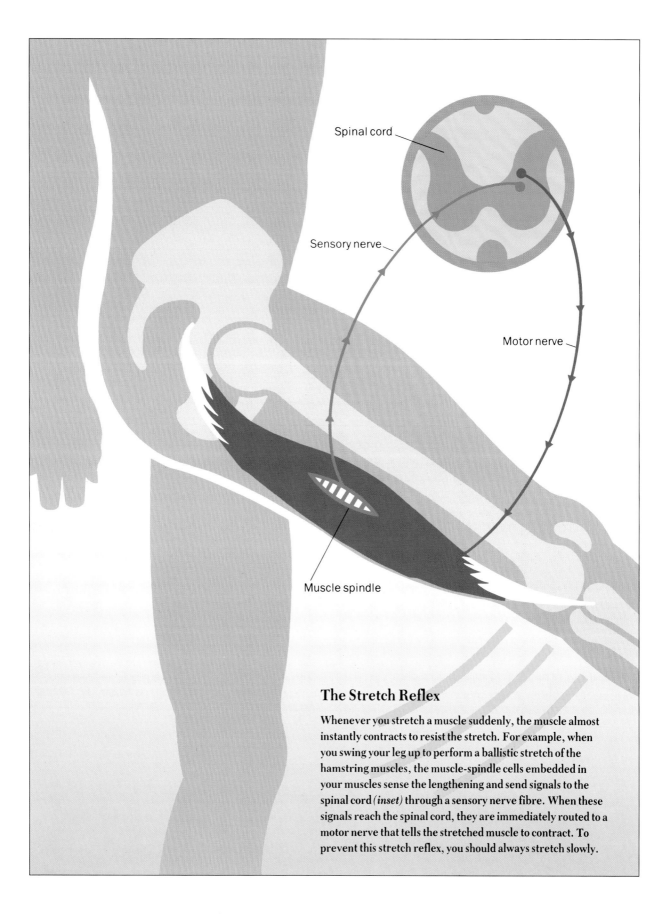

Spinal cord

Sensory nerve

Motor nerve

Muscle spindle

The Stretch Reflex

Whenever you stretch a muscle suddenly, the muscle almost
instantly contracts to resist the stretch. For example, when
you swing your leg up to perform a ballistic stretch of the
hamstring muscles, the muscle-spindle cells embedded in
your muscles sense the lengthening and send signals to the
spinal cord *(inset)* through a sensory nerve fibre. When these
signals reach the spinal cord, they are immediately routed to a
motor nerve that tells the stretched muscle to contract. To
prevent this stretch reflex, you should always stretch slowly.

reduces the chance of injury. Muscles that are short and restrict the natural range of motion in the joints are more susceptible to pulls, tears and stress injuries than those that are long enough to allow a full range of motion. Good flexibility also improves athletic performance. Short muscles detract from the grace of the gymnast, dancer and ice skater, may limit the muscular power of the golfer and tennis player, and may even lead to injury. Short calf muscles, for instance, can place undue stress on the foot, leading to a variety of orthopaedic problems, including painful Achilles tendinitis.

Flexibility is also crucial for correct posture, which in turn affects both your athletic performance and your general well-being. People who stand and sit correctly — their head centred, shoulders down and back, chest high and abdomen flat — give the impression of being alert and confident. Those who slump and have rounded shoulders, drooping head and excessive curvature of the spine — due to short chest, hamstring and pelvic muscles — may develop a poor self-image and convey an unfavourable impression to others.

Can a lack of flexibility cause health problems?

Lack of flexibility can create poor posture, resulting in mechanical imbalances in the back, hip and neck. These imbalances pull body segments out of line, causing stress, strain and even worse posture. The resulting muscular tension, joint strain, and ligament and cartilage damage can produce deformity. Short chest muscles and weak shoulders, for instance, cause rounded shoulders, which can lead to kyphosis (hunchbacked spine), a sunken chest and impaired respiratory capacity. Tight hip-flexor muscles and short hamstrings and back muscles can rotate the pelvis forwards, resulting in lordosis (excessive curvature of the lower back), chronic lower back pain and sciatica (a radiating pain in the thighs or buttocks along the sciatic nerve). Drooping your head forwards may produce headache, dizziness and chronic strain on the muscles at the back of the neck, leading to neck and shoulder pain.

How can you increase your flexibility?

Simply using your muscles will help lengthen them to some extent. For instance, you are usually least flexible when you get out of bed in the morning. Then, just by engaging in your normal routine and using your muscles to walk, sit and stand, you gradually gain flexibility throughout the day. The vigorous movement of exercise also helps: studies show that callisthenics, for example, increase flexibility. In general, athletes and people who work out regularly are more flexible than non-athletes and sedentary persons.

You can even increase flexibility, however slightly, by taking a hot shower (*page 8, box*). Warming connective tissue appears to increase its pliability: one study showed that by deep-tissue warming to 45°C, you can increase the range of motion in a joint by as much as 20 per cent. Cooling the joint to 18°C reduces flexibility by 10 to 20 per cent. These changes in flexibility are temporary, however. The preferred method of enhancing muscular flexibility is through a stretching programme.

Stretching to Run Well

Flexible calf muscles and ankles help you to run better. A well-stretched foot *(bottom)* can maintain contact with the ground longer than a stiff foot *(top)* — letting you push off harder with each running step you take.

Can a muscle stretch itself?

Muscles are like ropes: they exert force by pulling, not pushing. Similarly, muscles cannot lengthen themselves; they can only contract and relax. Most skeletal muscles are attached to one or more joints. When they contract, they move the joints. Therefore, stretching a muscle requires an external force, such as gravity or the contraction of an opposing muscle, to move a joint and stretch the muscle. Each of the exercises in this book uses such a force to achieve a stretch.

How much stretching is required to make a muscle more flexible?

To increase a muscle's length, studies show, you must regularly pull it about 10 per cent beyond its normal length: that is the point where your muscle feels stretched enough to be slightly uncomfortable but not enough to cause pain.

How often should you stretch?

The idea of lengthening a muscle in a progressive stretching programme to increase flexibility is related to the overload principle used to build muscle strength. To increase muscular strength, you must regularly contract the muscle against resistance with a slightly greater force than it is used to. In time, the muscle responds to the overload by becoming stronger. Similarly, to increase flexibility, you must regularly stretch the muscle slightly beyond its normal length. It will adapt to this overload by becoming longer, rewarding you with a greater range of joint motion. Studies show that you should stretch three to seven days a week to increase your flexibility. For maintaining flexibility, three days a week is probably adequate.

What are some of the immediate benefits of stretching?

Stretching is a natural, relaxing sensation. It helps relieve tension and the feeling of stiffness. Many people stretch in one way or another as soon as they get out of bed in the morning. Most people also stretch intermittently while sitting at a desk or driving a car for long periods of time. These simple routines do not increase general or long-term flexibility — they are simply pleasurable movements.

Stretching is not only pleasurable, it can also alleviate pain. For example, since one common cause of lower back pain is short, tight hip-flexor muscles, a stretching programme to lengthen these muscles may reduce the risk of lower back pain. Some experts think that stretching can help to prevent or alleviate the approximately 80 per cent of all cases of lower back pain which are caused by tightness and spasms in the musculature of the back and pelvis.

You can stretch to reduce muscle soreness associated with stress injuries, which result from overdoing sports and exercises. Ac-

Four Types of Stretch

Not all stretching techniques are equally able to lengthen muscles. Say, for example, that you want to stretch your chest muscle, which you use to swing your arm forwards. By swiftly swinging your arm backwards, the momentum forces the chest muscle to stretch. But this sudden ballistic movement induces the stretch reflex *(page 10)*, and your chest muscle contracts. As a result, a ballistic stretch allows your arm to swing only about 90 degrees (a). You can override the stretch reflex by swinging your arm back slowly. This sustained, or static, stretch increases the range of motion by a few more degrees (b).

You can increase a static stretch by using an external force, such as someone pushing your arm back, or by holding your hand against a wall and turning your body against the stretch (c). Most of the stretches in Chapters Two and Four rely on this technique. The longest stretch of all (d) is possible with a method called contract-relax, explained in Chapter Three. This technique entails briefly contracting the muscle to be stretched while a partner, a wall or any other external force prevents movement. As you relax, your limb can be pushed into an even greater stretch.

cording to one theory, this type of soreness is produced by a cycle of muscle tension, soreness and increased neural reflex activity, which results in more muscle tension and soreness. Slow, deliberate stretching reduces the neural activity in the muscles, thus breaking the cycle and reducing the pain.

What is the difference between a flexibility training programme and using stretches to warm up?

A flexibility training programme consists of stretching exercises designed to improve general flexibility when performed regularly. These exercises should work on muscle groups all over the body, concentrating on the tighter muscles. A flexibility warm-up is a group of stretches performed just before engaging in exercise or sports, and is designed to elongate temporarily the muscles directly involved in that activity. For instance, stretching out for running would involve working primarily on the hip flexors, quadriceps, hamstrings and calves. The warm-up routine is less extensive than the flexibility training programme and therefore less effective for improving general long-term flexibility. There is no evidence to suggest that sporadic flexibility warm-ups can result in long-term gains in joint range of motion such as those attained by a regular flexibility training programme. Stretching exercises as part of a sports warm-up, however, have been shown to increase a joint's range of motion by 4 to 18 per cent for 90 minutes or more. For more information on stretching routines designed for specific sports, turn to Chapter Four.

Is it dangerous to have too much flexibility?

Too much flexibility without muscle strength can cause instability in the joints, leading to dislocations and other traumas. Victims of poliomyelitis and other diseases or injuries of the neuromuscular system may suffer from this condition. However, it is unlikely that you can ever become so flexible from a stretching programme that you will have this problem. Nor will you become "double-jointed", a congenital condition that results in unusually flexible joints and permits contortions of limbs and torso.

Overly flexible or lax joints can result from stretching ligaments, the connective tissue that binds joints together. Ligaments, unlike muscles, are not elastic and therefore remain lengthened when stretched repeatedly. Weight-bearing joints such as the knee, ankle and hip may become unstable and susceptible to dislocation or abnormal twisting, resulting in injury. It is widely accepted among athletes that lax joints can lead to injury; many athletes therefore tape joints to increase stability. Most athletes who have lax joints also strengthen the supporting muscles in order to improve control over their joint flexibility. Their concern may be unwarranted, however, since studies do not show there to be a direct correlation between lax joints and frequency of athletic injuries.

S tudies show that stretching can help to relieve delayed muscle soreness after strenuous exercise. And evidence now suggests that stretching can at least reduce and sometimes prevent dysmenorrhoea, or painful menstruation. If you suffer from dysmenorrhoea which is not the result of a disease, you can probably relieve your symptoms by regularly performing stretching exercises of the muscles in the pelvic region.

Does weight training reduce flexibility?

Although it is commonly thought that muscle-bound people are inflexible, studies show that strength training, when done properly, does not limit flexibility. Body builders who regularly stretch their muscles as well as strengthen them have better-than-average flexibility.

What are the most important muscles to stretch?

Since flexibility is specific, you can increase a muscle's length only by stretching that particular muscle. Studies show, however, that people who stretch tend to stretch their longest muscles and neglect their shortest. The challenge, then, is to identify the muscles that are tight and to spend the bulk of your stretching time working on them, not on muscles that are already sufficiently flexible.

Generally speaking, the muscles most in need of stretching are the ones on which you place the greatest demands. Most reasonably active people should routinely stretch the following muscles: calves (to increase the range of motion in ankles and to prevent calf pain and Achilles tendinitis), hamstrings (to prevent running-related injuries), inner thighs (to reduce the chance of groin pulls), quadriceps and hip flexors (to prevent knee stiffness and lower back pain), and chest and shoulders (to prevent rounded shoulders and restricted range of motion).

Is it ever too late to get flexible?

One of the most obvious signs of advancing age is reduced flexibility. In far too many cases, range of motion becomes so severely restricted that an elderly person may be afraid of getting injured simply by walking or climbing stairs.

Luckily, inflexibility can be reversed, even among the elderly. In a study that compared the joint stiffness of a group of 20 young men (aged 15 to 19) and a group of 20 elderly men (aged 63 to 88), it was found that both groups could reverse joint stiffness with equal ease. A number of other studies have shown that virtually anyone, regardless of age, can improve flexibility by stretching.

I t is widely reported and commonly believed that tall, thin people are generally more flexible than those who are short and stocky. Although studies do suggest a direct relationship of total height and limb length to flexibility, the correlation is so slight that it is of little practical importance.

How to Design Your Own Programme

The simple tests on pages 18-19 will allow you to assess your flexibility. But even before you take the tests, ask yourself the questions here. You do not need to determine your flexibility level preeisely — you can often tell how supple your muscles are simply by using them and listening to their signals.

How Flexible Are You?

1 Can you touch your toes?

Touching your toes without bending your knees is the age-old test of flexibility. But, in fact, touching your toes tells little more than how flexible you are in the hamstrings and lower back. And, in order to keep you feeling good and safe from injury, flexibility must be a whole-body phenomenon. Some experts believe that the standing toe touch may be dangerous under certain circumstances because it can place stress on the lower back.

2 Can you sit with your legs outstretched and touch your head to your knees?

Most dancers can, but if you can, you may be trying too hard to become flexible. Forcing a stretch can lengthen ligaments as well as muscles. Muscles have extensibility and elasticity. When you stretch them, they spring back. Ligaments, however, are extensible but not elastic — they will not spring back. Once a ligament is stretched, it will stay stretched and may cause instability in a joint, especially in the hip, knee and ankle. Studies are not conclusive, but it appears that loose ligaments may lead to tears in cartilage and other soft tissue. Never try to force a stretch.

3 Do you often remind yourself to sit up straight and not slump?

If so, you should probably work on increasing the flexibility in your chest and shoulder muscles so that your posture while sitting and standing is more natural and less stressful.

4 Do you limp around the morning after a strenuous game of tennis or squash?

If your favourite sport makes you stiff the morning after, you should be working on increasing your flexibility. See Chapter Four for stretching routines specific to some of the most popular recreational sports.

5 Do you have leg cramps at night?

These are annoying but harmless. However, they probably indicate that you are overdue for a stretching programme. See Chapter Two.

6 Do you suffer from backache frequently?

Backache is among the nation's major health complaints; yet it could often be prevented simply by increasing flexibility. Good posture and strong, flexible muscles in the lower back and pelvis may help keep pressure off the discs in the lumbar region and so help prevent the condition that leads to herniated or ruptured discs. The illustration on page 21 will guide you to stretching routines for the back.

7 Do you play sports often?

If your answer is yes, then your flexibility may vary depending on the sport you play. Athletes in different sports, studies show, display different flexibility profiles. Athletics enthusiasts, for example, outperform wrestlers in certain tests. Furthermore, sports and exercise are selective in the muscles they lengthen. For example, hardly any sport improves the flexibility of inner-thigh muscles, and for athletes these muscles are among the most likely to get torn or pulled, usually from an abrupt lateral leg movement. So if you play sports often it pays to stretch regularly.

8 Do you do ballistic stretches?

That is to say, do you use vigorous bouncing, jerking or rocking movements to stretch your muscles? Since many athletic activities are ballistic in nature, some experts think that some ballistic stretching is good for you if you have already become generally flexible through static stretching exercises. And studies show that ballistic stretching is at least as effective as static stretching for improving flexibility. But there is great potential for pulling or tearing muscles with ballistic stretching, and most people should avoid it altogether.

Do You Get Cramps When You Work Out?

People who engage in sports or other strenuous activities often get muscle cramps. Usually the best way to prevent cramps is by stretching — both before and after exercise. If a cramp does occur, however, the best first aid is to stretch the muscle immediately. Gentle message also helps.

If the cramp recurs in the same place, it may be a symptom of a slight muscle tear — and a warning to ease up. But sometimes a muscle cramp is brought on by dehydration after prolonged exercise; the dehydration causes an imbalance in calcium, sodium or potassium. If this is the case, there is a simple solution: drink water before and during exercise. This will usually restore the correct mineral balance.

Measuring Your Flexibility

There is no best level of flexibility. Everyone has a different degree of flexibility that varies from limb to limb, from day to day, sometimes even from hour to hour. No single test can give you a sense of your overall flexibility. However, you can get a general assessment by testing the range of motion you can achieve in the major joints of your body. Furthermore, by taking a number of tests that measure specific muscles and muscle groups, you can determine where to concentrate the most effort.

Perhaps the greatest benefit of a flexibility test is to establish a baseline before beginning your training programme. You will then have a gauge by which to measure your progress. The five simple tests on these two pages measure flexibility in the lower back, hamstrings, hip flexors, shoulders and calves — areas where flexibility is particularly important among active people. All you need is a ruler and a box or step about 20 centimetres high. Ask a friend to help you take the measurements. Perform the tests about once a month to chart your progress. Remember that you are not in competition with anyone in achieving good flexibility. For the best results in this or any other fitness programme, you should proceed at your own pace.

Two of the muscle groups important to your overall flexibility are the lower back and hamstring muscles. To test their flexibility, sit with the soles of your feet against a box or step and your arms outstretched *(top)*. Reach as far forwards as you can towards the edge of the box without bending your knees. At the beginning of your flexibility programme, you may not be able to reach the box. Later, you may be able to reach as far as in the lower illustration. Get a partner to record how far your fingertips reach on a ruler extended 15 centimetres in front of the box's edge *(above)*. Rate your flexibility using the chart below.

How Far Can You Reach?
(in centimetres)

	Men	Women
Excellent	35+	37+
Very good	27-34	29-36
Fair	18-26	18-28
Poor	9-17	9-17
Very poor	8 or less	8 or less

Sit on a box or a straight-backed chair, holding your back erect. Rest one leg on the floor while extending the other. If your hamstrings are adequately flexible, you will be able to extend the leg fully without moving your other leg or altering your upright seated position.

While lying prone with one leg bent, get your partner to grasp your knee with one hand and, pushing down on your pelvis with the other, raise your leg. If your quadriceps and hip flexors are flexible, your partner will be able to raise your knee several centimetres without causing you undue discomfort.

Raise your right elbow and reach behind your back *(right)*. Place your left hand in the small of your back and slide it upwards. If you can touch your hands behind your back and overlap your fingers, your arms and shoulders are adequately flexible. To test your calf muscles, stand about a metre from a wall with your feet spread shoulder-width apart *(far right)*. Place your hands on the wall and bend forwards until your chin touches the wall. You should be able to do this while keeping your body straight and your feet flat on the floor.

Choosing
an Exercise

Once you have taken the flexibility tests on pages 18-19 and determined which of your muscles need improvement, you can use the illustrations on the right and opposite to select the most appropriate exercises in this book. You do not have to perform every exercise listed for each muscle group; one or two will usually be enough. But you can try each exercise to find the ones you are most comfortable with.

If you engage in another form of exercise or play sports and you wish to use stretching routines as part of your warm-up and cool-down, turn to Chapter Four. There you will find stretching routines for some of the most popular recreational sports.

The dynamic movement routines in Chapter Five are stretches that work the body as a whole, rather than isolating specific muscles and muscle groups. Therefore, the illustrations on these pages do not refer to those routines.

Whichever exercises you choose, be sure to read the following four pages in order to perform the exercises safely and effectively.

NECK
Pages 52, 53, 71, 74, 75

SHOULDER
Pages 73, 75, 87-89, 91-93

CHEST
Pages 48, 49, 68-70, 73, 85-93

BICEPS
Pages 48, 68, 69, 91

OBLIQUES
Pages 39, 84-86, 91

ABDOMINALS
Pages 39, 44, 91

WRIST
Pages 82, 83, 85, 87

HIP FLEXORS
Pages 40-45, 64, 66, 82, 83, 88-93

GROIN AND INNER THIGH
Pages 36, 37, 43, 62, 63, 80, 82, 84-86, 89, 93

QUADRICEPS
Pages 40, 41, 44, 45, 64, 65, 81, 88, 89, 93

SHIN
Pages 41, 50, 82, 83, 85

ANKLE AND FOOT
Pages 50, 51, 86

UPPER BACK
Pages 48, 49, 70, 71, 86, 87

LATISSIMUS DORSI
Pages 46, 73, 82, 84, 86, 91

TRICEPS
Pages 49, 68, 69

SPINE
Pages 35, 70-73, 85

LOWER BACK
Pages 30, 31, 34, 35, 60, 61, 63, 71, 80-82, 86, 89

BUTTOCKS
Pages 31-34, 60, 71, 81-83, 92, 93

OUTER HIP AND THIGH
Pages 32, 33, 66, 67, 81, 82, 85, 89

HAMSTRINGS
Pages 30, 31, 33, 35, 38, 39, 58, 59, 61, 71, 81, 89, 93

CALF AND ACHILLES TENDON
Pages 30, 31, 46, 47, 58, 59, 80, 82, 83, 85, 87-93

Common Mistakes

Relax When You Stretch

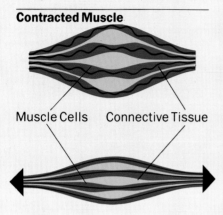

Contracted Muscle

Muscle Cells   Connective Tissue

Relaxed Muscle

When you try to stretch a contracted muscle *(top)*, as in performing ballistic stretches, proportionately more of the external force is placed on the muscle fibre than on the connective tissue. This may result in microscopic tears. When you stretch a relaxed muscle *(above)*, you stretch the connective tissue, which helps prevent injury.

A growing body of research suggests that some people who stretch to avoid injury when they work out or play sports can get injured from the stretches themselves. In one survey of 4,000 running injuries, stretching exercises were found to be a major cause of injury. The study also determined that those who were injured performed certain exercises that placed excessive stress on joints, ligaments and muscles. The most common of these are shown opposite. If you avoid these stressful stretches and observe the following precautions, you will be able to design a safe stretching programme.

Perform slow static stretches, not bouncing or ballistic stretches such as leg kicks. Although studies show that ballistic stretches are as effective as static stretches for increasing flexibility, there is a possibility that you will rupture ligaments and cause microscopic tears in your muscles. One reason for this is that bouncing causes the muscle to contract at the same time as you are forcing it to stretch. Also, ballistic stretches are not as deliberate as static stretches, and the uncontrolled momentum of your limb may overload a joint and force it to move beyond its natural range of motion, very probably damaging the connective tissue.

Stretch your muscles only about 10 per cent beyond their normal length. When a muscle is stretched to this limit, you should feel a comfortable tightness in the centre of the muscle. Do not stretch any farther; if you feel discomfort at the muscle's end attachments, you are stretching too far and subjecting the tendon to too much tension. Never stretch to the point of pain. And remember that improving your flexibility is progressive — it cannot be done in one session. Forcing your muscles to stretch beyond their capability will cause injury and also loss of elasticity.

Always work within a joint's natural range of motion. If you force a joint to move beyond its natural range of motion, you may rupture or overstretch the ligaments. This can occur with certain dangerous stretches that place most of your body weight on one particular joint. Both the "plough" and the "hurdler's stretch" shown opposite can place excessive stress on certain joints. Deep knee bends can overstretch ligaments in the knees. Also, a ballet barre stretch can place a great deal of force on the extended knee, possibly damaging the cartilage and ligaments. This stretch can also compress the sciatic nerve, causing pain to radiate down the back of the legs from the buttocks.

Stretch both before and after a strenuous workout session. A single stretching session will significantly improve flexibility and joint range of motion for at least 90 minutes. Stretching beforehand may reduce your chance of injury and improve your athletic performance. However, some athletic activities may tighten your muscles or cause delayed soreness. By stretching afterwards, you can regain flexibility and prevent soreness.

If you do happen to become injured from overstretching, treat the injury like any other stress injury. Reduce the intensity of your exercise and apply ice packs to the affected area. Ice will lessen the discomfort and reduce the swelling. Of course, if you experience severe pain or if the discomfort of an injury lasts for several days, consult a doctor.

The plough *(left)* is a popular but dangerous stretch for the hamstring and back muscles. It places tremendous pressure on the back of the neck, which must support your entire body weight.

Toe touching with locked knees *(below)* is all too common as a stretch of the lower back and hamstrings. These muscles must contract to support your body at the same time as you are trying to stretch them. Not only is toe touching inefficient as a stretch, but it can also result in injury.

Ballistic stretching, such as kicking your leg with the knee locked *(above)*, will stretch your muscles. But it will also induce the stretch reflex. This type of stretching often causes delayed localized muscle soreness.

The hurdler's stretch *(left)* should not be performed by anyone except very flexible athletes. The awkward twisting can cause strain and torn ligaments in the bent knee.

The Training Regimen

Training your muscles to stretch farther is similar in concept to training them for strength: you must use the overload principle. Just as the only way to strengthen muscles is to exercise them slightly beyond their normal capacity and then progressively increase the workload, so to increase their flexibility you must follow a progressive stretching programme.

As you advance in a flexibility programme, you will not see steady improvement from one day to the next. Muscle soreness, motivation, ability to relax, room temperature and warm-up preparation are among the factors that influence your range of motion. But regardless of your flexibility at any particular time, by following the guidelines here you should notice an improvement in a month.

HOW HARD

Studies show that you should stretch a muscle about 10 per cent beyond its normal length in order to increase its flexibility. At this point, you should be stretching about as far as you can without feeling pain. If you do feel pain, consider it a warning to ease up on the stretch.

HOW OFTEN

You should stretch at least three days a week in order to obtain minimum benefits. For optimal results, however, you should stretch four to seven days a week.

HOW LONG

Most experts agree that you should hold a stretch for between 10 and 60 seconds to lengthen a muscle effectively. For the best results, however, you should stretch a muscle or muscle group for 15 to 30 seconds, pause and then repeat the stretch once or twice.

Special Situations

If you spend long periods sitting or standing, or if you are so busy during the day that you do not have time for a full workout, you can benefit from the following exercises.

SITTING

When you sit a lot, tension builds up in your lower back, shoulders and neck. Sitting for extended periods of time can also shorten your hamstrings and hip flexors and cause soreness in your buttocks. This set of exercises will counteract tension and discomfort in these areas. Half of them can be done while you are sitting.
- Hamstring stretch on a stool, page 31
- Buttocks, pages 32-33
- Hip-flexor stretch on a stool, page 43
- Seated back stretch, page 35
- Seated chest, back and shoulder stretches, page 49
- Neck stretches, pages 52-53

STANDING

The strain of prolonged standing is usually felt in the muscles of your feet, calves, hips and lower back. These exercises are performed standing upright, and you can do them at any time, anywhere.
- Foot and shin stretches, pages 50-51
- Calf stretches, page 47
- Hamstring stretch on a stool, page 31
- Hip-flexor stretch, page 42
- Chest stretch against a wall, page 48
- Full-body circle for the sides, shoulders, hips and back, pages 114-115

QUICK STRETCHING

If your time is limited, doing only a few stretches is better than doing none or trying to hurry through a full routine. Here is a round-up of stretches that you can complete in five minutes.
- Calf stretches, page 47
- Hamstring stretch on a stool, page 31
- Hip-flexor stretch against a wall, page 43
- Roll down for back, hips and neck, pages 98-99
- Full-body circle, pages 114-115
- Diagonal reach for the shoulders, sides and inner thigh, pages 108-109

Ten Guidelines for Stretching

1. **CHOOSE THE BEST TIME OF DAY.** Find a period when you are not likely to be interrupted by phone calls or other distractions. Proper stretching requires concentration and patience. Be sure that you do not rush through your routines. Also, do not work out immediately after a meal; a full feeling will make you uncomfortable.

2. **WEAR LOOSE-FITTING CLOTHING.** Special exercise outfits are not essential for a stretching programme, but you should wear loose, comfortable clothing that does not restrict your movement. To achieve the best results, you should stretch on a carpeted floor in bare feet. For comfort's sake, do not wear a belt or jewellery.

3. **WARM UP.** Perform a five to 10-minute aerobic warm-up, such as jogging on the spot or stationary cycling, before you stretch. You will be adequately warmed up when you begin to sweat. Warming up helps to increase the circulation and temperature in your muscles, which in turn increases their pliability. Stretching muscles that are cold is less effective than stretching them when they are warmed up.

4. **LISTEN TO YOUR BODY.** Remember that your flexibility changes from day to day and you may not be able to perform on one day the stretch that you did the day before. Never try to force a stretch; instead, ease into it and take the muscle only to the point of slight discomfort. The stretch should always occur in the centre of the muscle, not at the attachments, and should never cause pain.

5. **BREATHE EVENLY.** The key to stretching is to remain relaxed during your exercises. Breathing rapidly or irregularly or holding your breath may make you tense. Instead, go into a stretch as you are exhaling, then concentrate on breathing normally and slowly.

6. **BE SPECIFIC.** Flexibility does not diffuse itself throughout the body. Achieving flexibility in part of the body, or having stretched a particular muscle, does not mean that you will necessarily gain flexibility in another area. Be sure to pay special attention to those body areas that are the least flexible and stretch them more often.

7. **DO STRETCHES IN PAIRS.** Work for bilateral flexibility — that is, equal flexibility on both sides of your body. When stretching one side of the body, be sure to follow with the same stretches on the other side.

8. **PROGRESS AT YOUR OWN SPEED.** Do not attempt to force your muscles into flexibility. Begin slowly and gradually work towards your goals. Never try to compete with another person by seeing who can stretch farther. Flexibility is an individual matter.

9. **TAKE EXTRA TIME IF NECESSARY.** If you have been inactive for a while and your muscles are unaccustomed to being stretched, then you should start slowly. The same is true if you have muscle soreness as the result of a stress injury from overdoing a sport or exercise. However, never stretch muscles that are torn or strained; you will only worsen the condition.

10. **KEEP TRACK OF YOUR PROGRESS.** Test your general flexibility *(pages 18-19)* at the beginning of your training programme to establish your flexibility baseline. Then retest your suppleness monthly as you progress. Once you have achieved the flexibility you want, continue stretching about three times a week to maintain your level.

CHAPTER TWO

Basic Stretching

A whole-body routine for greater flexibility and better posture — any time, anywhere

Static stretching, also known as sustained or passive stretching, is by far the most popular technique for improving flexibility. It is safe, convenient and pain-free. You can perform static stretches whenever and wherever you want. You can do them standing up, sitting or lying down. And you do not need a coach, a trainer, exotic exercise equipment or a health club. All that is required for most static stretches is loose, comfortable clothing, a wall or other solid surface to lean against and, for some stretches, a chair or bench to support you.

One of the great advantages of static stretching is that it helps you to become better acquainted with the interrelationships of your body's muscles and tendons. Its slow, deliberate movement teaches you to feel how your muscles work in groups. You will become more aware of muscle tension, contraction and relaxation; and you will be able to isolate particular muscle groups to determine which groups are tighter or less flexible than others. By recognizing the limits of your muscles' flexibility, you can avoid overstretching and injury; furthermore, you will be better able to gauge the improvement in your flexibility.

Static stretching involves a slow pull that extends a muscle just beyond its normal length. Continued pressure holds the muscle in a stretched position for a sustained period. To benefit from static stretching, you must hold the stretch for at least six seconds. However, to get the best results, you should hold a stretch for 15 to 30 seconds and then repeat the exercise once or twice. The stretching must be forceful enough to enhance flexibility but not so rigorous as to cause injury to the muscles or tendons. Most experts agree that you should perform static stretches to the point of mild discomfort but never stretch so far that you feel acute pain. While stretching can help alleviate muscle soreness, it can also cause soreness when overdone. If you are just starting a stretching programme, therefore, you should be especially careful that you do not overstretch a muscle.

Because a static stretch is gentle and prolonged, the technique reduces the muscle-spindle stretch reflex, which would normally cause the muscle to contract when it is stretched *(page 10, box)*. For this reason, mild static stretches are superior to forceful ballistic stretches, in which a person bounces or swings part of his or her body to gain momentum and force a stretch. Ballistic stretching causes the muscle spindles to induce a reflexive contraction in the very muscle you are trying to stretch. As long as your stretch is slow and deliberate, however, you can safely lengthen a muscle beyond its normal reach as you develop flexibility.

Static stretching is most effective when you can apply an external force to aid your stretch. As the stretching exercises on the following pages show, there are a number of ways to do this. For example, you can induce a static stretch of your chest muscle simply by drawing your arm as far back as possible and holding it there. But that stretch is limited by the flexibility of your chest muscle and by the strength of the opposing muscles on the other side of the shoulder joint pulling your arm back. The weaker those muscles, the less effective the stretch. You can get a much better stretch of the chest muscle by bracing your hand against a wall and twisting your body away from the wall. Then you do not have to rely on the strength of your chest's opposing muscles; instead, your leg and trunk muscles can apply greater force by using the wall for leverage. You will be able to hold the stretch longer without the opposing muscle becoming fatigued.

Another way to introduce an external force to enhance static stretching is to apply the leverage of one or more limbs against that of another. You can, for instance, support yourself against a wall or lie face down on the ground and grasp your ankle, pulling it towards your buttocks. This technique will stretch your quadriceps on the front of your thigh far more effectively than if you tried to stretch them by contracting your opposing hamstring muscles and lifting your foot without external assistance.

Getting Started: the Elongation Stretch

A simple and easy stretch that will help you release muscular tension is the elongation stretch, shown above. You should precede every stretching session with this exercise. Lie face up on the floor, stretching your arms out and bringing your legs together. Extend your arms and legs as far as you can, pointing your fingers and toes out, your palms facing the ceiling. Tilt your pelvis so that the whole length of your spine makes contact with the floor. Tuck your chin in. Hold this stretch for about 10 seconds, then relax. Repeat three times.

The elongation stretch is a full-body routine: you should feel the stretch in the top of your feet, your ankles, shins, abdominals, chest, sides, shoulders, lower back, upper back and arms. When performing the elongation stretch, be sure to breathe deeply and slowly. Shallow or rapid breathing can cause muscular tension.

Gravity, too, can play a role in stretching. When you lean into a wall with one or both legs extended backwards, gravity pulls your body down and applies force to the musculature of your lower leg, thereby stretching your calf muscles.

When you embark on a static stretching programme, give yourself plenty of time to stretch. Do not hurry through it. Be sure you are properly supported so that you do not lose your balance. Too often, for instance, people try to perform a quadriceps stretch by pulling their heel back to their buttocks while trying to balance on one foot. Stretching in this manner not only causes undue muscular tension in the supporting leg, but the unsteady stance can diminish the effectiveness of the stretch.

At the beginning of your stretching programme, you may notice inappropriate contractions, chiefly in the opposing muscles. For instance, while stretching your hamstrings you might feel a tense quivering or tightening of the quadriceps. These muscle contractions are normal. Some people embarking on a stretching programme also report a temporary numbness in some muscles while they stretch them. As you gain experience and develop better flexibility and control, both the contractions and the sensations of numbness should disappear; your muscles should feel a warm tightness as they are being stretched and a pleasant looseness afterwards.

Hamstrings

A group of three large muscles in the back of the thigh, the hamstrings are among your body's most important muscles, since they act to straighten the hip and bend and rotate the knee. Virtually every sport and physical activity makes use of these muscles, and, as a result, they are frequently subject to tightness and stress injuries.

In the stretching routines that follow, many of the exercises are shown for only one side of the body: for example, in the hamstring stretch on the right, the left leg is being stretched. When you do this or any other exercise that stretches muscles on either the right or the left, be sure to repeat the exercise for the other side of the body.

Sit on the floor with one leg extended and the other leg bent at the knee. Loop a towel round your foot and pull your leg. This is a good stretch if you have particularly tight hamstrings and calves.

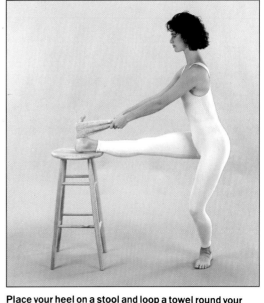

Place your heel on a stool and loop a towel round your foot. With your standing knee bent, pull your leg into the stretch. Be sure to keep your back straight.

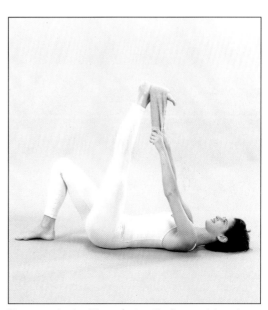

Lie on your back with one foot on the floor and the other leg extended in the air. Loop a towel round the foot of your extended leg and draw your foot towards you as far as you can.

Sit on the floor with one leg extended and the opposite knee bent. Keeping your back straight, lean forwards slowly to grasp your toes. This will stretch your hamstrings, lower back and calf muscles.

Buttocks

The buttocks region is composed of nine major muscles. They include the gluteals, which straighten the hip, rotate the thigh and take part in straightening the knee. Because the buttocks muscles stabilize the pelvis, they are particularly active while you walk. They can become strained with overuse, and they can tighten with inactivity. To prevent inflexibility in the buttocks muscles, you should perform at least one of the exercises on these two pages regularly.

Extend your left leg and cross your right leg over it *(above)*. Draw your right knee back with your left arm. For a greater stretch, tuck your left foot under your right thigh *(below)*.

Stretch the muscles in your right buttock by lying face up on the floor, resting your right ankle just above your left knee and drawing your left knee towards your chest by pulling with both hands *(above)*. Then stretch the hamstrings as well as the buttocks by extending your left leg *(above, right)*.

Lying on your back with your arms outstretched, twist your hips to the left and tuck your right calf under your left knee *(above)*. The weight of your left leg will help stretch the right buttocks muscles. For a hamstring stretch *(above, right)*, straighten your left leg and extend the right leg; try to bring your toes to your left hand.

Lower Back

Sit on the floor with your legs crossed, then twist to the right and lean forwards on your hands, stretching the lower back *(above)*. To stretch the lower back and buttocks, lean forwards and bring your forearms towards the floor *(below)*.

The muscles and connective tissues of the lower back support your upper body. Like the rigging on a ship's mast, the deepest layers of muscles anchored in the lower back rope up the entire spine and attach to the vertebrae. The latissimus dorsi — the muscle you use when you pull your elbow back — also attaches to the lower back region. No wonder, then, that the lower back is frequently the site of muscle and connective-tissue stress. Poor posture, of course, can exacerbate lower back pain. To relieve pain and reduce stress to the region, perform these stretches.

Sit on a stool or a chair with a high seat. Gently drop your body towards your lap, letting your hands dangle to the floor and your head drop between your legs.

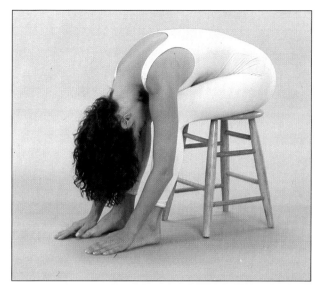

Lie on the floor, bend your knees and bring your feet towards your head. Hold on to your feet and pull your knees towards your chest to stretch your lower back and hamstrings.

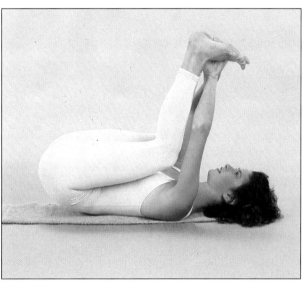

Kneel down and place your hands on the floor with your elbows extended and your back straight. Arch your back like a cat.

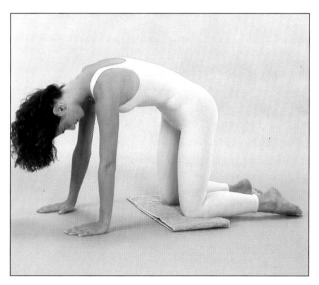

Inner Thighs/1

The muscles of the inner thigh and groin area are called the adductors, since they adduct the thigh, or move it in towards the opposing leg. The adductors are connected to the lower portion of the pubic bone and run down the inside of the thighbone, where they attach along a tendinous strip. Many people who exercise regularly ignore their inner thigh muscles, allowing them to become short and tight. These muscles can then be easily injured, resulting in what are commonly called groin pulls. To reduce the chance of injury and to extend the range of motion in your legs, you should routinely stretch your inner thigh muscles with the exercises here and on pages 38-39. Most men have more difficulty than women in attaining the positions shown. Do not strain to achieve them; greater flexibility will come with time.

Lie on your back with your knees bent outwards and spread as far apart as comfortable. Prop your feet on a wall for support and press down on your knees.

While lying on your back, extend your feet in the air and spread your legs as far apart as you can. Press down on your inner thighs with your arms.

Draw one knee up and support it with your hand as you straighten your other leg, where you will feel a concentrated stretch.

Bring the soles of your feet together and grasp your feet with your hands. Pull your feet towards you to stretch the inner thigh muscles closest to your groin area.

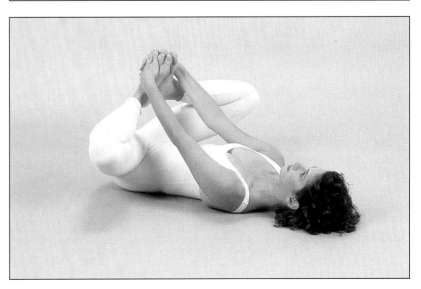

Inner Thighs/2

With your legs stretched in front of you, straighten your knees and spread your legs as wide as you can. To stretch both the inner thigh muscles and the hamstrings, lean forwards and rest on your elbows *(right)*. To concentrate on the musculature in your right leg, rotate your torso to the right and reach towards your foot with your left hand *(far right)*. Then lean to the left and raise your right hand towards the ceiling to stretch the abdominals, obliques and other side muscles *(below)*.

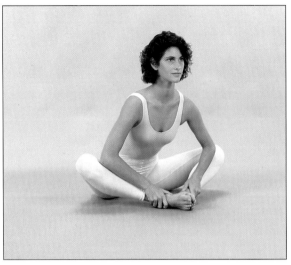

Sit on the floor with the soles of your feet together. Grasp your feet and lean forwards, pressing your forearms on your shins.

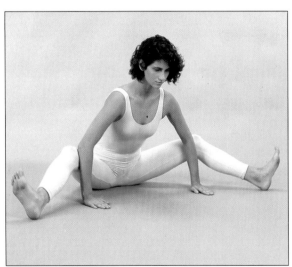

While still sitting, spread your legs as far apart as you comfortably can, keeping your knees bent. Lean forwards from the waist and place your hands on the floor. Press against your knees with your elbows.

38

Quadriceps and Hip Flexors/1

The quadriceps are four thigh muscles that begin on the hipbone and the thighbone and become united on a single tendon that is attached to the kneecap. These muscles work together primarily to straighten the knee. The hip flexors are a group of muscles, including one of the quadriceps, which lift your thigh. Tight quadriceps and hip flexors can limit your ability to run and jump. In addition, tight hip flexors can tilt your pelvis forwards and lead to lordosis, or excessive curvature of the lower back.

Lie on your stomach and grasp your right foot with your right hand. Pull your heel to your buttocks to stretch the quadriceps *(above)*. To stretch the hip flexors, pull your knee off the floor *(below)*.

Lie on your left side and grasp your right foot with your right hand *(above, left)*. Pull back on your foot until you feel a stretch of the quadriceps and hip flexors. Lie face up on an exercise table with your left leg tucked towards your chest, grasping the knee with your left hand *(above, right)*. Extend your right leg over the edge of the table. Pull on your foot with your right hand. To stretch the hip flexors and shin muscles, stand facing away from a stool. Using a wall for balance, rest the top of your right foot on the seat *(right)*. Bend your left knee until you feel the stretch.

Quadriceps and
Hip Flexors/2

Take an exaggerated step forwards with your
right foot. Brace yourself on your right
knee and extend your left leg backwards to
stretch the hip flexors.

Kneel on your left leg with your right foot flat on the ground, turned out at the same angle as your right shoulder. To increase the stretch and include the right inner thigh, lean farther over your right foot.

Perform a lunge stretch by using a wall for balance. Place your palms against the wall and extend your right leg behind you to stretch the hip flexors.

Place your right foot on the seat of a stool for a lunge variation. The higher the stool, the greater the stretch you can achieve. Grasp your shin and lean forwards to lengthen the hip flexors in your left leg.

Quadriceps and
Hip Flexors/3

Kneel and lean backwards on your hands *(above)*. Be sure to keep your body straight and do not drop your pelvis. You will feel this stretch in all the muscles in the front of your thighs. Extend your right hand towards the ceiling *(below)* to add an abdominal stretch.

With your hands on the floor for balance, extend your left foot behind you while keeping your right foot on the floor; lower your chest towards your right knee *(above)*. This is a difficult stretch if you do not have flexibility in your hip flexors.

Kneel on your right knee and place your left foot flat on the floor. Balancing on your right hand, twist round to hold your right foot with your left hand *(above)*. Pull your foot upwards to stretch the quadriceps as well as the hip flexors.

45

Calves

Your calf muscle is composed of two distinct parts, the gastrocnemius and the soleus. The gastrocnemius is the large bulging muscle of the calf. It is connected to the Achilles tendon and is principally involved with lifting the heel off the ground and pushing off for walking, running and jumping. The soleus extends underneath the gastrocnemius and also connects to the Achilles tendon. Not as powerful as the gastrocnemius, the soleus pulls on the ankle joint when you stand on your toes.

Many people, especially runners, have inflexible calf muscles. Tight calves can result in Achilles tendinitis, pronation, or inward roll of the foot, and plantar fascitis, an inflammation of the connective tissue in the sole of the foot.

Stand with your legs slightly apart. Bend forwards from the hips and place both hands on the floor, stretching the calves. Your heels may rise slightly.

Place your palms against a wall, drawing your left knee forwards and extending your right leg behind. Keep your right knee locked and your heel on the ground to stretch the gastrocnemius *(top, left)*. To stretch the soleus, flex your right knee slightly *(top, right)*. Lean into the wall with both feet extended behind you and both knees locked to stretch your left and right gastrocnemius muscles *(above, left)*. Flex your knees slightly to include a soleus stretch in both legs *(above, right)*.

47

Upper Body

Stretching exercises for the upper body are important not only to protect you from muscle strain, but also to improve your posture and general appearance. Tight or weak chest and shoulder muscles, for instance, may result in rounded shoulders and bad posture, which are aggravated by sitting hunched over a desk all day. The upper body stretches on these two pages will help to alleviate muscle tension in your chest and shoulders. You can perform the stretches on the opposite page while sitting at a desk.

Stand erect with your feet together. Grasp the ends of a towel with both hands and hold the towel behind your head *(right)*. This is a general stretch of the chest, shoulders and upper arms.

Face a wall and bend from the hips so that the top of your head points to the wall. Place your palms against the wall for a stretch of the shoulders and arms *(above)*.

Sit upright in a straight-backed chair. Twist to the right and hold on to the chair frame. Pull back with your left arm and hold tight with your right to stretch your upper and middle back muscles.

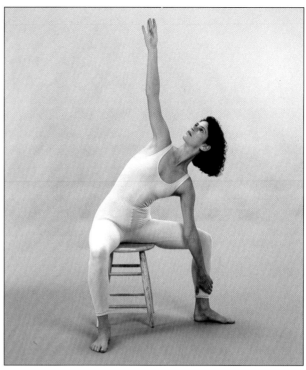

Sit on a stool with your legs spread apart. Grasp your left calf with your left hand. Stretch your right hand towards the ceiling to elongate your chest and upper and middle back muscles.

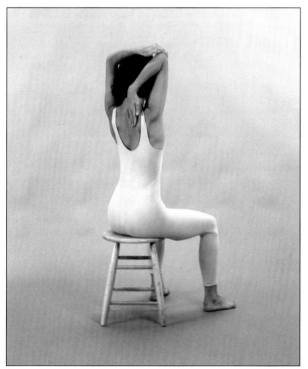

Sit upright with the palm of your right hand behind your neck. Grasp your right elbow with your left hand and pull it towards the back of the head, stretching the triceps of your right arm.

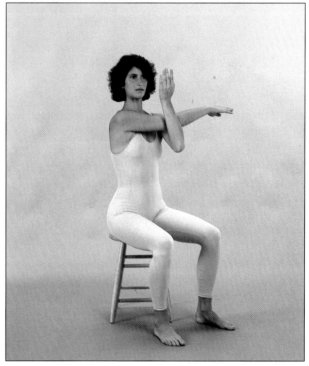

Sit on a stool and swing your right arm across your chest. To enhance a stretch of the right triceps and shoulder, place your arm in the bend of your left elbow and pull up with your left arm.

Feet

The foot is an amazingly complex structure that not only provides the strength to support your entire body, but also imposes subtle yet significant changes in pitch and direction to control your posture and gait. A well-functioning foot routinely absorbs tremendous force. Walking, for instance, subjects the foot to a force of up to 120 per cent of your body weight with each step. Running subjects the foot to even greater loads — up to about five and a half times your body weight.

For all that the foot must do, it requires remarkably little care. Shoes that provide support and shock absorption are all that your feet normally need. In addition, stretching your feet helps to increase circulation and relax the musculature.

Sit comfortably in a chair with your foot off the floor and follow this sequence: first extend your toes as far as you can, feeling the stretch from your ankle to your toes along the top of your foot *(right)*. Then turn your foot in *(far right)* to stretch the muscles along the outside of your foot. Pull your toes back towards your shin so that you feel tightness along the sole *(below, left)*. Finally, turn out to lengthen the inside muscles *(below, right)*.

Kneel on the floor. Lift your right knee and draw it forwards slightly *(opposite)*. Press the top of your right foot to the floor. This stretches the muscles of the metatarsal region, your ankle and shin.

Neck

Not counting the larynx, your neck contains more than 30 muscles that act to rotate your head and to flex forwards, backwards and from side to side. In addition to giving you this mobility, your neck must also protect your spinal cord and support your head. In daily living, these functions can sometimes be at odds, resulting in neck strain and stiffness. Regular exercise that requires extensive neck movement, such as cycling or swimming, can also cause neck strain. You can help to prevent this problem by performing the exercises on these two pages. When using your arms to assist movement, take special care not to jolt or strain the neck.

Gently drop your head backwards to extend your neck. Do not force your neck back, but let your head drop naturally to lengthen the muscles along the front of your neck.

Grasp the back of your head with your right hand, and pull it forwards and to the right to stretch the trapezius.

Place your right hand over your left ear, and pull your head to the right. This will stretch the mastoid muscle.

Interlace your fingers behind your head. Push your chin to your chest to lengthen the muscles in the back of your neck.

CHAPTER THREE

Partner Stretching

Not only fun, but more effective

Partner, or assisted, stretches involve two people: one person stretches and the other person helps to achieve the stretch. Assisted stretches can increase your range of motion farther than static, single-person stretches. The reason is simple: for most of the static stretches covered in Chapter Two, the muscle-stretching force is provided by body weight — applying the force of one limb on another or grasping an immovable object for leverage and then pulling. All these forces are limited by gravity or by your own strength. More effort and leverage can be applied to your limbs by a partner, increasing the length and duration of a stretch.

Partner stretching also allows you to perform a type of stretch called contract-relax. To carry out a contract-relax stretch, you must first perform a static stretch. Your partner holds the stretched limb in place while you push as hard as you can against the stretch with an isometric contraction. Then you release the contraction while your partner pushes your limb to a new point of tightness. You will find that this stretch is greater than that which you can normally achieve. Although the contract-relax technique can sound complicated in theory, it is actually quite simple in practice *(opposite, box).*

The contract-relax method of stretching has consistently proved more effective than traditional techniques. In one study, Swedish researchers asked two groups of subjects to stretch three times a week. One group used the ballistic method and the other the contract-relax technique. After 30 days, the researchers discovered that the contract-relax group had improved its flexibility more than twice as much as the ballistic-method group. The improvement in joint range of motion for those using the ballistic method averaged between 1.4 and 3.5 degrees, while improvement among those using the contract-relax technique averaged between 6.0 and 10.5 degrees.

In an American study comparing the contract-relax method with both ballistic and static stretching, subjects were randomly assigned to one of four groups: ballistic, static, contract-relax or control (no stretching at all). After a six-week, three-times-a-week flexibility-training programme, the subjects were tested for flexibility of their shoulder, trunk and hamstring muscles. The results confirmed the Swedish tests, indicating that contract-relax techniques are superior to other stretching methods for improving flexibility.

Physiologists developed the contract-relax method as one of a group of therapies for paralysed individuals. The doctors called this group of therapies proprioceptive neuromuscular facilitation, or PNF. Although a number of studies have documented the effectiveness of PNF techniques for lengthening muscles and increasing the range of motion, researchers do not agree on why this is so. The most widely accepted theory concerns the Golgi tendon organs, which are nerve fibres that sense tension in muscle tendons. During the contraction phase of the PNF routine, the tension caused by the strong pull of the isometric muscle contraction induces the Golgi tendon organs to send signals to the central nervous system. These signals, called inhibitory impulses, are part of a protective reflex response to prevent muscle and tendon tears. The inhibitory impulses override any signals from the muscle spindles to contract the muscle further. Then, when the muscle is stretching during the relax phase, the inhibitory impulses dampen the stretch-reflex response of the muscle spindles *(page 10).* Although the neuromuscular process is complicated, the simple result is that you can stretch farther.

An added benefit of the contract-relax method is that it increases strength. According to one recent study, PNF stretching can be superior to weight training for improving athletic performance. Researchers randomly assigned 30 women students to one of three groups — a PNF group, a weight-training group and a control group. After training the women three times a week for eight weeks, the scientists found that the PNF group performed significantly better than either the weight-trained or the control group in both throwing and jumping abilities. Those women who trained with PNF exercises

The Contract-Relax Method

To perform a contract-relax stretch, the basis for most of the routines in this chapter, your partner first guides you into a conventional static stretch. As you begin to feel the stretch, you reverse the motion and push against your partner as hard as you can. This is the contract phase, which is shown on the right, top, for a stretch of the hamstring muscles. When you push against your partner, who provides immovable resistance, be sure to use only the muscles you are going to stretch. For example, in the hamstring stretch, you push with your thigh — which requires keeping your leg straight — not with your calf.

After five or six seconds, relax your muscles completely. Your partner then pushes the muscles back into a stretch that extends them farther than before. The two of you hold this position, shown on the right, bottom, for 20 to 30 seconds.

improved their throwing distance by 25 per cent and their vertical-jump ability by 16 per cent, while the weight-trained group had increases of only 12.8 and 9.9 per cent respectively. Many athletic coaches consider contract-relax routines an important component of their training programmes.

Some contract-relax exercises can be performed without a partner. You can, for instance, stretch your inner thigh muscles by sitting cross-legged on the ground, pushing upwards with your knees against the palms of your hands for the contract phase, then relaxing your inner thigh muscles and continuing to push down with your hands. But most PNF routines require another person to provide adequate isometric resistance during the first stretching phase and then strength to push you into the new stretch. The following pages offer a number of partner-assisted stretches, most of which involve the contract-relax method. Be sure to choose a partner who is sensitive to your needs and aware of your level of flexibility. He or she should stretch your muscles gently, until the stretch becomes slightly uncomfortable, but not so that it causes pain.

Hamstrings and Calves

Your hamstrings, among the longest and strongest muscles in your body, are likely to become tight and inflexible if you do not stretch them regularly. This is also true of your calves, which form part of a biomechanical pulley system with the Achilles tendon, the heel and the plantar fascia along the bottom of the foot. The contract-relax method of stretching can be the most effective way to loosen the hamstrings and the calves. You can perform either the contract-relax stretch or a simple static stretch lying with your back on the ground, on a cushioned massage table or even on top of your kitchen table, putting a towel underneath you for comfort.

As in the previous chapter, any stretch that works muscles on one side of your body should be repeated for muscles on the other side.

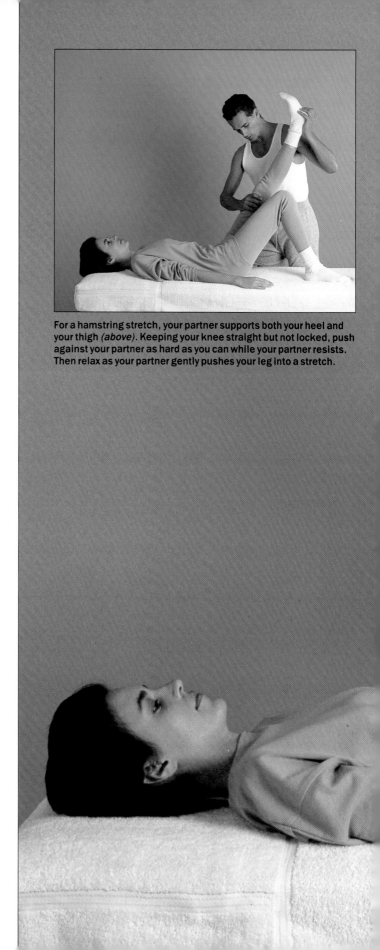

For a hamstring stretch, your partner supports both your heel and your thigh (above). Keeping your knee straight but not locked, push against your partner as hard as you can while your partner resists. Then relax as your partner gently pushes your leg into a stretch.

To perform a calf stretch, lie on your back with your knees flexed and your feet flat. Straighten one leg as your partner grasps your heel and draws it towards the ceiling. Push your leg against this stretching motion, then relax as your partner eases your leg into a new stretch.

Hamstrings and Lower Back

Since the hamstrings attach to the lower part of the pelvis, they frequently influence the lower back region. Tight hamstrings can tilt the pelvis and lead to an inflexible lower back. It makes sense, then, to stretch not only the hamstrings but also the lower back region. The partner-assisted stretches here will help to ease tightness in your lower back as well as to increase the flexibility of your hamstrings.

Sit cross-legged with your hands at your sides. Your partner kneels behind you and places her hands on your back *(top)*. Push against her, then reach forwards to stretch *(above)*. This position stretches your lower back and some buttock muscles.

To stretch your lower back and hamstrings simultaneously, sit on the floor and either keep your hands at your sides or grasp your toes *(inset)*. Push against your partner. Then relax, dropping your head and elbows as your partner pushes you gently into the stretch *(above)*.

Inner Thighs

Many people — especially men — have tight inner thigh muscles, which can be particularly troublesome for those who are physically active. Recreational runners, for instance, often suffer from pulled groin muscles. The inner thigh muscles, like the hamstrings and the muscles of the lower back, are attached to the pelvis.

Sit cross-legged with the soles of your feet together. Your partner places her hands on top of your knees while you attempt to push your knees upwards. As you relax, your partner presses your knees gently towards the floor for the stretch *(above)*.

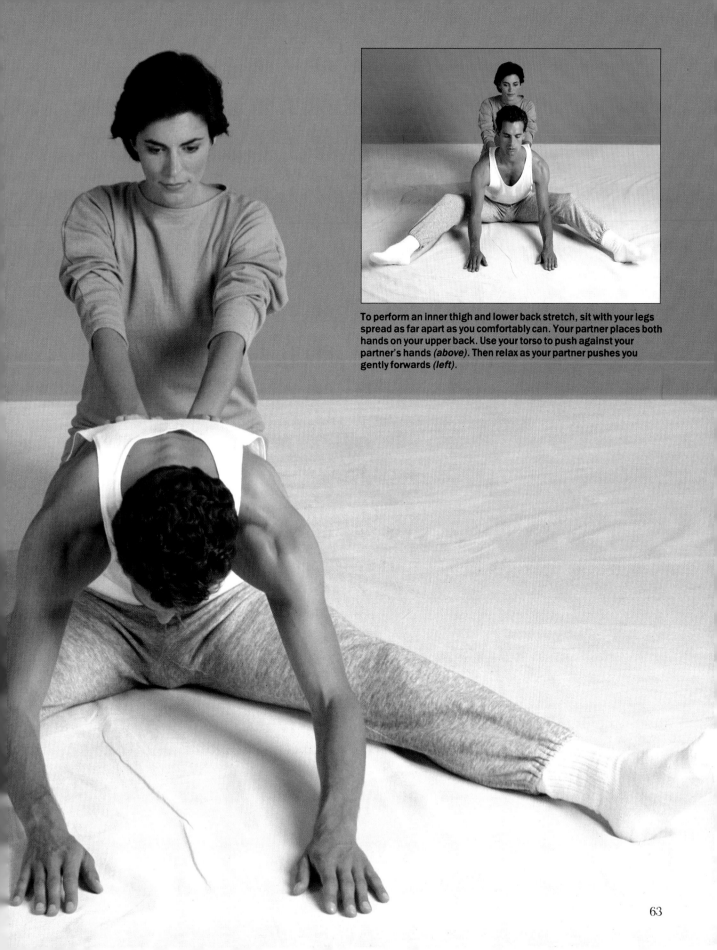

To perform an inner thigh and lower back stretch, sit with your legs spread as far apart as you comfortably can. Your partner places both hands on your upper back. Use your torso to push against your partner's hands *(above)*. Then relax as your partner pushes you gently forwards *(left)*.

Quadriceps and Hip Flexors/1

The quadriceps and hip flexors are the primary muscles along the front of your thigh. They are extremely powerful and therefore lend themselves particularly well to partner-assisted routines, since your partner can use your leg as leverage.

If you run, cycle or climb stairs frequently, you should also stretch the iliotibial band, a strip of connective tissue that runs from one of the hip flexors on the outside of your hip all the way down to the outside of your knee. The iliotibial can become tight from these activities and cause a burning sensation round the knee. The stretch on pages 66-67 is designed to loosen the iliotibial band.

To isolate your hip flexors, lie face down on a table as your partner presses one hand against your right pelvis, grasps your right leg just above the knee and lifts it into a stretch *(above)*.

To perform a quadriceps stretch, lie face down on the floor or a massage table. Your partner stabilizes your pelvis with one hand and bends your leg with the other. Attempt to straighten your knee by pushing against her hand, then relax as she bends your leg to a new point of tightness.

Quadriceps and
Hip Flexors/2

For an additional hip-flexor stretch, lie on your back with your buttocks near the end of a table. Stretch your right leg out and draw your left leg up *(left, top)*. Your partner helps hold your left leg in place as you extend your right leg. Relax as your partner pushes your right leg down and your left knee towards your chest *(left, bottom)*.

To loosen the iliotibial band, lie on your side at the end of a table. Bend the bottom leg to support your pelvis but keep your other leg straight. Your partner uses one hand to hold your pelvis and the other hand to press down lightly on your knee *(right)*.

Chest

The stretches shown on these two pages will increase flexibility in your pectoral, or chest, muscles; they also involve some muscles in the shoulders and arms. People with weak and inflexible shoulder and chest muscles frequently display poor posture: they slump and have rounded shoulders. These contract-relax exercises should help correct those conditions. As always, your partner should exert gentle force and check that you are suffering no discomfort.

Lie face down on a table. As your partner draws your arms up by the wrists, the force of your body weight stretches your chest muscles. Keep your elbows loose.

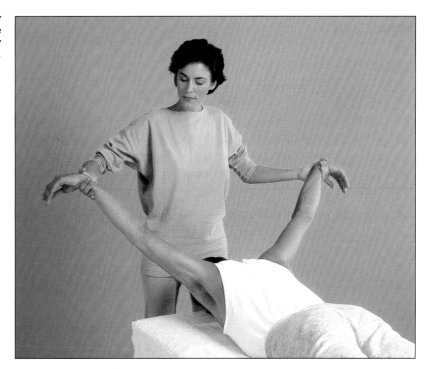

Sit cross-legged with your back supported by your partner's leg. Interlace your fingers behind your head. Your partner pulls your elbows back.

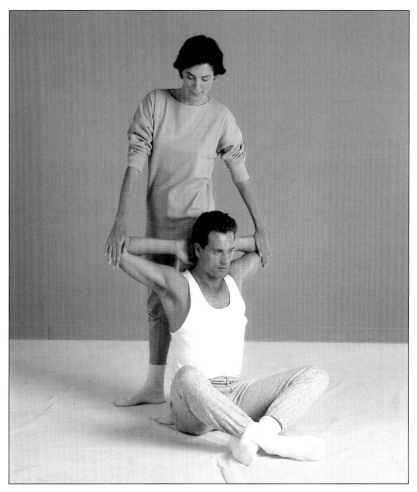

Lie face down on a table with your hands clasped behind your head *(opposite)*. Your partner grasps your elbows and draws them up. You will feel a stretch of the pectorals of the chest, and the biceps and triceps of the upper arm.

Back

Your back contains dozens of muscles in five crisscrossing layers. The outer layer consists of the latissimus dorsi and the trapezius, both of which influence shoulder movement. Most of the inner layers of back muscles are anchored on your pelvis and are connected to your vertebrae and ribs. These muscles hold your spinal column erect and permit your spine to move in all directions; they allow you to rotate round and arch backwards, forwards and sideways. Despite their importance, these muscles are often too short and easily strained, causing backache. Partner-assisted back stretches help provide gentle traction and stretch these deep spinal muscles.

To stretch the muscles of the upper back and chest, kneel and extend your hands in front of you while pressing your chest downwards. Your partner overlaps her hands and presses gently on your spine.

To stretch the entire spine, assume a kneeling position, lean over and sit back on your heels. Your partner places her hands on your head and lower back. Without moving her hands, she exerts pressure gently but firmly in opposite directions *(above)*.

To stretch the lower back, buttocks and hamstrings, lie on your back and draw your legs up. Your partner grasps your ankles and pulls them over your head *(top)*. She must not pull your knees over your head, lest too much weight rest on the back of your neck. To stretch just the lower back and buttocks, your partner pushes your knees to your chest *(above)*.

Gentle Traction

Physiotherapists have long recognized the importance of traction, which helps to mobilize a joint by separating the two opposing joint components. Traction can also contribute to easing muscle tension, increasing blood flow, encouraging a greater range of motion and relieving pressure on nerves. Although professionally supervised traction using weights of 5 to 35 kilograms can reduce compression of the vertebrae, it can also lead to overstretching and muscle spasm. Gentle traction, such as the exercises shown here and on the following two pages, is a safe, pleasant way to relax your muscles and reduce intervertebral pressure.

For back traction, lie face up with your hands over your head, your knees flexed and your feet on the table. Keep your elbows loose and slightly flexed as your partner uses his body weight to pull gently on your arms.

Your partner can also provide gentle traction for your legs and pelvis. Lie face down on the table so that he can grip your ankles and lean backwards *(above)*.

To stretch the back, chest and shoulder muscles, lie face down on the table. Keep your elbows slack as your partner gently pulls you forwards *(top)* and from side to side *(above)*.

Neck Traction

Lie on your back with your arms at your sides and your feet flat on the table *(below)*. Your partner gently cradles your head in her hands and pulls back and up slightly, lengthening the muscles in the back of the neck. She can also turn your head to each side and, supporting your head with one hand, push gently against your shoulder to stretch the muscles at the top of your shoulders *(above and left)*.

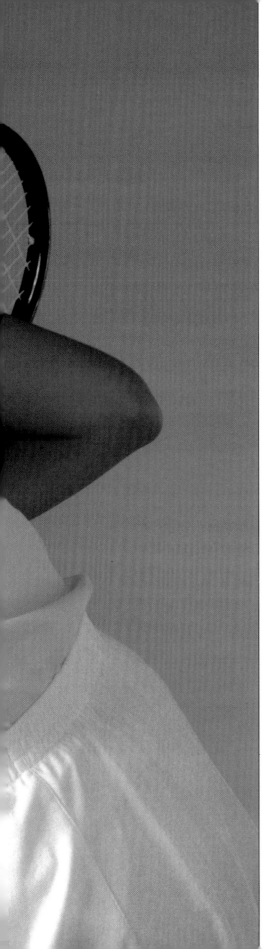

CHAPTER FOUR

Stretching for Sports

*Better performance,
fewer injuries*

To most athletes, the benefits of stretching and good flexibility are obvious. A full range of motion in certain joints is necessary for the successful performance of many sports. Dance, figure skating and gymnastics, for example, require extensive muscular flexibility and a good range of motion in virtually all body joints. Contact sports such as football, hockey, basketball and rugby also require a better-than-average range of motion in the joints, as well as flexibility in the muscles of the thigh, hip flexors, trunk, arms, shoulders and neck. For most non-contact sports such as athletics, swimming and golf, you need varying degrees of flexibility specific to the particular sport. For example, swimmers who perform the front crawl will especially benefit from improved flexibility in the rotator cuff muscles of the shoulders. Without it, they may experience limitations in their stroking ability and possibly develop a stress injury called swimmer's shoulder.

Flexibility is also related to power. Experiments have shown that muscles can store elastic energy and then release that energy in a powerful burst. The more a muscle can stretch, the greater its potential for energy release during contraction. Thus, muscle elasticity is important for sports that require forceful stretch and contraction, such as jumping and throwing. Javelin throwers, for instance, need to be especially flexible in the chest. Like the string of a bow, the major chest muscle is pulled taut as the arm swings back to throw the javelin; like an arrow, the farther the javelin is drawn back, the more force can be applied to it and the greater its velocity when released.

Runners, too, may be able to improve their performance by increasing their flexibility. According to the U.S. Olympic track coach, tight muscles present internal resistance to movement. Runners with loose, pliable leg muscles, therefore, may be able to move their legs faster and longer than those with tighter muscles. And by adding just two centimetres to your stride length through stretching, you can gain about 15 metres per kilometre. For such distance events as a 10,000-metre run or a 26.2-mile marathon, even a minuscule increase in stride length can make the difference between a world-class performance and simply finishing the race.

Coaches and athletes alike generally accept the importance of stretching and flexibility for the enhancement of sports performance. Although few studies have been conducted in the area of flexibility and performance, there is some evidence that increased flexibility can improve performance in certain specific activities such as long jumping, ball hitting, throwing and sprinting. No studies have established minimum norms of flexibility necessary for each sports activity, however; nor has research determined how general sports performance may change in response to a progressive stretching programme.

While it is clear that some level of flexibility is essential for the successful performance of any sport, once you have reached that level, you may not be able to improve your performance further by continuing to increase flexibility. For example, slight variations in flexibility among a group of top gymnasts will not determine who will rank highest in competition. However, gymnasts and other athletes must stretch to achieve the level of flexibility required by their sport, and continue stretching to maintain that flexibility.

Some studies suggest that stretching can also help prevent injuries. A study of Swedish football players showed that athletes with muscle tightness and restricted range of motion have a higher-than-average incidence of injuries. Muscle strains occurred in 31 per cent of the players with muscle tightness, but in only 18 per cent of the players with normal flexibility. Studies in the United States show that those players with tight or inflexible hamstring muscles may develop lower back and knee injuries.

The reason for this is that muscles adapt to exercise by shortening to the range of motion habitually used in the exercise. And vigorous ex-

Hand Stretches

Your hands are crucial tools for playing almost any sport. First, they translate muscle power from your body into the motion of a racket, ball or club. They must also control that motion, giving a precise arc to a basketball, for instance, or the right angle and velocity to a tennis shot. In addition, your hands may have to support your body, such as during a long cycling trip.

Use the four simple exercises on the right to stretch your hands for power and flexibility. The top two are for your thumbs, the bottom two for your fingers. Before you perform them, shake your hands vigorously to increase circulation. Be careful not to force any of these movements.

Firmly but gently stretch your thumb towards your wrist. Do not force it.

Stretch your thumb in the opposite direction by pulling back on it.

Stretch your palm by pulling back on all your fingers at the same time.

Spread your fingers and pull them back one at a time.

ercise places greater loads on inflexible muscles, leading to chronic stress injuries. A short gastrocnemius muscle in the calf, for instance, may result in pronation, or inward rotation of the foot, which is the most common cause of stress injuries to the foot and can lead to ankle and leg injuries and even a stress fracture.

If you do get an injury, stretching may help you to recover more easily: it has been shown to reduce muscle soreness, and many athletes believe that it also speeds recovery. In addition, muscle injury often results in the formation of scar tissue, which is inelastic and acts to reduce a muscle's pliability. Thus, stretching exercises can help restore flexibility to an injured muscle.

Since flexibility is muscle-specific — that is, you become more flexible only in the muscles you stretch — and each sport places its own pattern of stress on joints and other body parts, your stretching routine must vary according to which sports you play. The following 14 pages offer stretching routines for some of the most often played recreational sports. These routines will not necessarily make you a better player, but they can keep you from getting injured and enhance your enjoyment of the game.

Sit on the floor and bend your left leg so that your left sole is against your right inner thigh. Bend forwards from the hips, using a ball for support. This stretches the inner thighs and lower back.

To stretch your calf muscles, keep your toes straight and your heels on the ground as you lean forwards.

Basketball and Football

Basketball and football are sports that require not only co-ordination and agility, but a great deal of stamina, jumping ability and speed. Both are fast games that involve sudden turns, dashes and leaps. In addition, both unavoidably involve occasional collisions.

Basketball and football players need strength and flexibility, particularly in their hips, thighs, calves and trunk. These two pages present six basic stretches that will help loosen you up to play either game. These stretches focus particular attention on the hip and knee regions, which are where most of the stresses of basketball and football playing occur.

While sitting, draw one knee up. Extend your arms and lean forwards from the hips to stretch the hamstrings of the straight leg.

Remain seated and cross your legs, pulling your right knee towards your chest. You will feel the stretch in your right buttock.

Lie on your right side and extend your right arm. Pull your left foot towards your buttocks but keep your knee in line with your hip to stretch your quadriceps.

Lie on your back with your arms outstretched. Twist your legs to the right. Cross your right leg over your left to stretch the outer hip, thigh and lower back.

Cycling

Lie on your back and extend your legs in the air, keeping your knees straight. Support your legs with your hands and separate them to stretch the inner thighs.

Lie on your right side with both arms extended as shown. Draw your left leg back until you feel a stretch in the hip flexors, outer thighs and latissimus dorsi.

Lie on your back and draw your right knee towards your chest. Use your arms to pull the back of your knee. You should feel a stretch in the hip flexors and lower back.

Cycling is an endurance sport that requires as much effort and stamina as long-distance running. As in running, the great muscles of the calves and thighs provide most of the driving force needed to propel you forwards. Cycling requires particular flexibility and strength in the hip flexors to draw the pedals up and, similarly, in the quadriceps to push the pedals down. For this reason, good cyclists often have unusually powerful and pliable thigh muscles.

Because cycling places such a demand on the musculature of the legs and trunk, endurance riding all too often leads to muscle strain and pain in the lower back. These discomforts occur in novices and seasoned cyclists alike. In addition, cyclists often suffer from neck stiffness and sore wrists. For neck soreness, turn to pages 52-53 and 74-75; otherwise, the five stretches presented on these two pages should be all you need to help you maintain flexibility for cycling.

Find an object just below waist level for support. Clasp your hands behind your head and place one foot on the object *(opposite)*. Keep your back straight and your heel on the ground to stretch the hip flexors, calf, Achilles tendon, chest and buttocks. Perform the stretch in the inset for the wrist flexors, shins and ankles. With your wrists reversed, lean forwards as shown: bending your right knee will stretch the ankle and shin in your left leg extending behind.

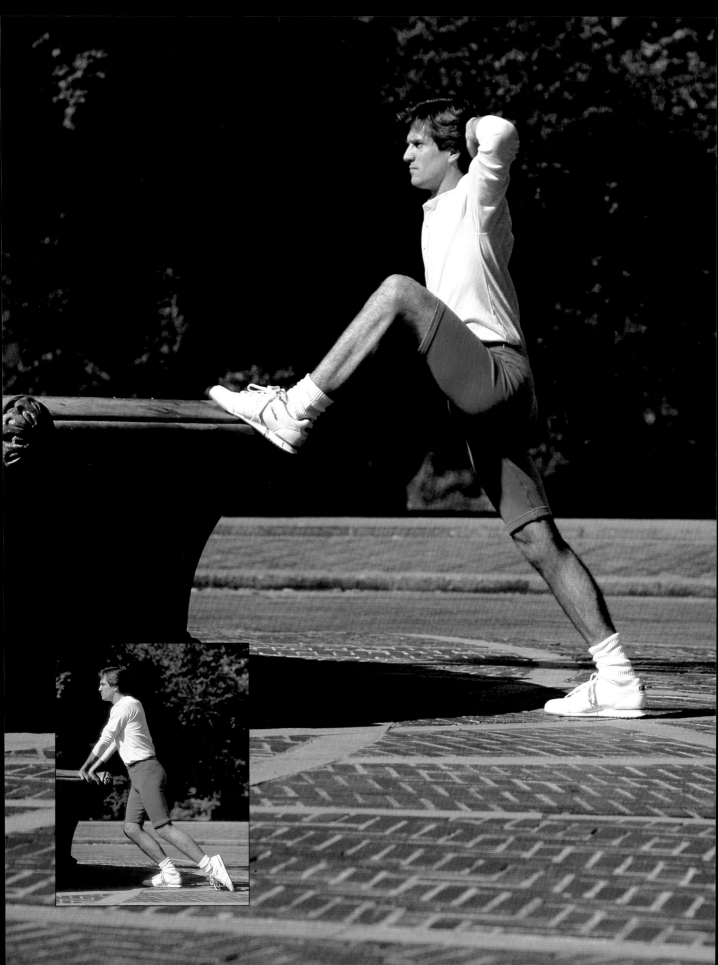

Golf

Golf is a popular weekend sport; yet most people tend to neglect the fitness aspects of the game. Golf requires a good deal more strength and endurance than most golfers realize, especially for those who carry their own golf clubs. Many weekend golfers also fail to appreciate the importance of fitness for improving their game and preventing injuries. A good golf swing involves a powerful twist of the arms, spine and shoulders in order to bring the head of the club round with sufficient force. In addition, the momentum of the club carries the golfer's arms into a wide arc, which may cause strains and even tears in the muscles of the shoulders, back, sides and wrists.

To minimize the chance of injury, and to give yourself the greatest range of motion in the joints of the shoulders and upper body, perform these four stretches.

Place your palms against a wall with your fingers pointing down. Move one leg forwards while keeping the other leg straight. Lean into the wall. This not only stretches your calf, Achilles tendon and wrist flexors, but should also help you to avoid golfer's elbow, an inflammation of the connective tissue in the elbow.

Turn sideways to a wall and support yourself with your left arm. Swing your right leg behind your left and lean on the outside of the foot, twisting your body to produce a stretch in the left side of your chest. This will also stretch the outer muscles of the right leg.

To improve flexibility in your spine, place your golf club behind your back and under the inside of your elbows. Then turn your head to the right and twist your body to the right from the waist up.

Extend one leg to the side and rest it on a bench or stool *(opposite)*. Grasping your golf club at each end and holding it above your head, bend sideways towards the extended foot. You will be stretching the latissimus dorsi, the obliques and the inner thigh of the opposite leg.

Racket Sports

Racket sports, which include badminton, squash, racketball and tennis, are excellent all-round conditioners. However, these sports are performed most frequently by recreational players who pay little attention to the fitness aspects of the activities. Most players launch straight into their games with little or no warm-up, play intensely for a short period of time and then stop playing abruptly, only to resume days or weeks later. The consequence is almost inevitably injury. Few realize how physically demanding these sports can be, or how much their game could improve if they simply took a little time to get into better condition. One of the best ways to improve your condition and to avoid unnecessary injuries is to improve your flexibility.

Racket sports require speed and agility, particularly for quick lateral movements. Thus, players with tight muscles may experience frequent groin-muscle pulls. And since returning a ball in play often calls for sudden lunges and stretches, pulls in the back, sides, wrist, ankles and shoulders are also common. These two pages offer five stretches to help you improve your racket game.

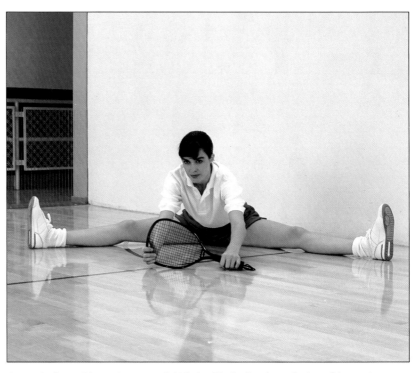

Sit on the floor with your knees straight but not locked and your feet as wide apart as comfortably possible. Hold your racket on the floor in front of you for support; lean forwards from the waist. You should feel a stretch of your inner thighs, lower back and upper back.

To stretch your chest muscles, stand at arm's length from a wall and place one palm on the wall as shown. Turn your body slightly away from the wall but keep your hand in place.

Grasp both ends of your racket and hold it over your head. Spread your feet apart and arc your body to the left, bending your right knee slightly but keeping your left leg straight.

To stretch your shoulder muscles, your
chest and spinal rotators, hold the racket
behind you and twist from the waist up.

Support yourself against a wall with the
backs of your hands, which will promote
flexibility in the wrists. Keeping one leg
straight will stretch the calf muscles as well.

Running

Running is probably the most efficient way to get into shape. Almost anyone can run at almost any time and with a minimum of expense. Studies show that virtually anyone can increase cardiovascular fitness with running, including children, the elderly and even heart-attack victims.

Running, however, places great stress on the body's muscles and tendons. According to one survey, about half a sample population of runners reported a running injury in the previous year that was serious enough to make them reduce training, take medication or see a health professional. A disproportionate percentage of running injuries occur among beginners who have not developed adequate strength or flexibility.

To avoid injury and increase your range of motion for running, thereby promoting a more fluid running style, you should perform the stretches on these two pages.

Sit on the ground and draw your left knee up. Lean forwards from the hips and reach for your right ankle to stretch the hamstrings of the straight leg.

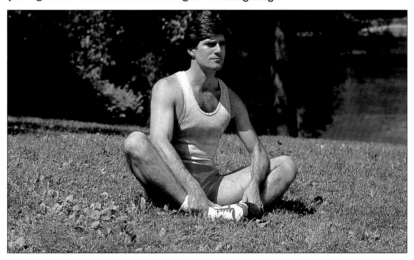

Draw the soles of your feet together and clasp your ankles for support. Lean forwards slightly from the hips to stretch your inner thighs and lower back.

To stretch the quadriceps, hold on to an object for balance, pull your right heel back towards your right buttock and keep your knee pointing towards the ground (left). Stretch your hip flexors, calves, shoulders and chest by clasping your hands behind your back and placing your left foot on an object about 30 centimetres off the ground. Keep your right knee straight, lean forward and pull your arms up (inset).

Lie on the ground with both legs extended. Bend your left knee and cross it over the right leg. Pull your knee towards the ground to stretch the muscles of the outer hip and thigh.

To stretch your chest, hip flexors and calves, face
a wall with your arms extended over your head.
Bend one knee and press your chest to the wall.

Swimming

Although you do not have to be particularly skilful or fit to enjoy swimming, this activity can place a tremendous demand on virtually all of your body's major muscle groups. Swimmers need strong arms, shoulders, chests and abdomens, since the muscles grouped in those areas provide the most stroking power. Because swimming is a dynamic sport that requires a full range of motion, particularly in the shoulders, swimmers must stretch out frequently to avoid tight muscles. Perform the six stretches on these two pages at least once a day.

Lie on your stomach and extend your arms, keeping your hips on the floor. You will feel the stretch in your abdominals and hip flexors.

Stand with your arms above your head and grasp your left elbow with your right hand. Pull your arm to the right *(top left)* to stretch the latissimus dorsi and obliques. For your shoulders and biceps, grasp a towel behind your back and pull it up with both arms *(top right)*. You can then use the towel to stretch the shoulder's rotator cuff muscles. Hold it behind your back and pull down with one arm while the other arm is just behind your head *(right)*. Then pull up with one hand over your head while the other is bent behind your back *(far right)*.

Volleyball and Netball

Volleyball and netball are games conducted at a fast pace and both require frequent bursts of speed.

Volleyball players need flexible shoulders and calves for spiking — smashing a ball downwards from the top of a jump. Netball players likewise need flexible shoulders for passing and defending.

For volleyball players, supple hip flexors and inner thighs are important so as not to pull a muscle when dropping down under the ball for a dig. Netball players need hip flexors that are supple as well as strong in order to stabilize the body during sudden accelerations and halts.

To stretch the hip flexors and buttocks, perform a lunge *(left)*. You may hold on to an object such as a railing for support. For chest and shoulder muscles, grasp a railing behind you and lean forwards *(inset)*. Place your right heel near the wall and bend your left knee to stretch your calves. Point your feet straight ahead and keep your heels down. Make sure to avoid jerky movements.

Spread your feet apart, bend one knee and drop towards the floor. Grasp a railing behind you with both hands and pull forwards to stretch your chest, shoulders and inner thighs.

Lie face up, keeping your back flat by raising your left knee. Pull back on your right ankle for a quadriceps stretch.

Sit on an exercise bench with one leg extended flat along the bench to stretch the hamstrings. Be sure to keep your back straight.

CHAPTER FIVE

Dynamic Movement

*A whole-body routine for fluid motion
in three dimensions*

In recent years, a new type of exercise called dynamic movement has evolved, blending ancient Eastern arts of movement with modern-day understanding of biomechanics, musculoskeletal anatomy and neuromuscular physiology. Its reinterpretation of the lilting, dancelike forms of Tai Chi and the deliberate actions of Yoga is aimed at enhancing body awareness, freedom of movement, co-ordination and flexibility, and providing release from muscular tension.

From the perspective of dynamic movement, most conventional stretching seems a one-dimensional activity. The action is most often an up-and-down or back-and-forth motion perpendicular to the body, and it ordinarily stretches a specific muscle or muscle group for a particular activity. Recommended stretching exercises for runners, for instance, elongate the muscles that get the most use: the calves, hamstrings and hip flexors. Sometimes, to add a second dimension, the athlete will stretch the muscles opposing the most-used muscles.

For the runner, these muscles are primarily the quadriceps along the front of the upper thigh.

Practitioners of dynamic movement think that this kind of stretching ignores a vital third dimension, the muscles that support the body as it moves. In daily life, they point out, we rarely move with the machine-like angularity implied by the one or two-dimensional hamstrings-quadriceps stretching routine. Even the simplest action often requires the simultaneous involvement of numerous joints and the action of dozens, even hundreds, of muscles. Fluid body movement, therefore, can occur only as a result of intricate teamwork among groups of muscles acting sequentially.

Almost every movement involves properties of dynamic movement. Even if you try to stand still, your body does not remain motionless but sways slightly over a stationary base. Try as you may, you cannot stay absolutely still. Experiments show that people tend to faint when they are held absolutely still. Therefore, swaying slightly aids circulation and ensures continued consciousness. In order to continue this slight swaying yet not lose control, the body oscillates round a centre line of gravity. Muscles and muscle groups all over the body alternately contract and relax. Even if you assume different positions or hold an object such as a book or a tray, your body automatically compensates and continues its oscillation. In dynamic movement, therefore, postural balance is seen as a fluctuation between stability and mobility.

Dynamic movement uses the stabilizing muscles that, when contracted, improve body stance and eliminate excessive movement that might occur as a body part moves. A stabilizing muscle keeps the area round it from moving so it can act as a fulcrum for other muscles to stretch and contract. This stabilizing action also prevents injury that might be caused by straining or by excessive stretching or compression of a joint. If you stand and then raise your right knee, the muscles most involved in lifting your knee are the right hip flexors. But the muscles that wrap round your right thighbone, for example, are also engaged, acting to guide the action and eliminate undesired rotary movements in the hip. The muscles in your trunk, pelvis and straight leg act to stabilize your body by alternately contracting and relaxing to maintain a position. While you are in motion, this type of force and counterforce occurs constantly in muscles all over your body, not just in the muscles most involved. It is impossible to understand running, for example, by viewing it simply as an action of the hip flexors, hamstrings and calves. It is a whole-body activity.

Exercise that involves the extra dimension provided by dynamic movement takes your body through various motions to lengthen and strengthen the supporting and assisting muscles. The first practitioners of dynamic movement, who were active in the 1920s and 1930s, used their exercises as a treatment to correct posture and alignment of the spine. In recent years, other disciplines such as sports medicine and Yoga have enhanced the exercises, and practitioners in

The Kinesphere: the Body's Field of Movement

The body operates within a three-dimensional space. From a standing position, you can reach upwards and downwards, sideways and forwards, backwards and diagonally. You can also twist and turn round in the opposite direction. The space within your reach has length, width and depth. That space can be perceived as a sphere of movement, called the kinesphere.

Unlike most traditional stretching and exercise routines, dynamic movement makes use of the entire space within your kinesphere. As you perform the dynamic movement routines shown on the following pages, you will become more aware of how your body movements function within this three-dimensional mode, not just in an up-and-down and back-and-forth action. Dynamic movement helps you to realize your body's full, complex ranges of motion and the interrelationships of its various parts.

the field now work mainly with dancers to help them gain greater spatial awareness through an understanding of body movements. There are several schools of dynamic movement, each named after its founder; the best-known are Alexander, Laban and Feldenkrais. But although techniques vary from school to school, all of the exercises — including the ones in this chapter — are concerned with moving through combinations of lying, sitting and standing. Ultimately, the feelings produced by dynamic movement are those of ease and efficiency.

To begin your dynamic movement routines, find a well-ventilated room, free from obstructions, where you will not be interrupted or distracted. It should have a floor covering such as carpeting or matting to prevent discomfort while you are lying down. Set aside plenty of time to perform your dynamic movement routines; performing them hurriedly will destroy the sense of fluidity you are trying to develop.

Wear clothing that is appropriate for any type of stretching: loose-fitting, non-binding leotards or exercise outfits are perfect. Whatever you choose, do not wear a belt, which would restrict your movement and could become uncomfortable, or shoes, since there is no jumping activity that would pose a risk of foot injury.

Preparing to Move

To get the most out of the dynamic movement exercises here and on the following pages, try to quiet your mind. Think of nothing but the physical act of moving. Never hurry through a movement or force yourself to attain a particular position. Do not perform a series of repetitions of the exercises rapidly, as if they were callisthenics; instead, move through an exercise slowly, with the poise and concentration of a dancer. Do each sequence two or three times during a session; before long they will become familiar and relaxing.

When you are performing a dynamic movement routine, be sure to breathe normally and rhythmically. Start each session by taking several deep breaths to help relax your entire system, and keep breathing at a moderate pace. You should never force your breathing or constrict it.

As with more traditional stretching techniques, you should work both sides of your body equally. A routine that involves moving your body in one direction should be repeated in the other direction.

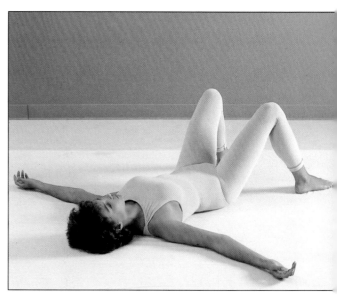

Double-Arm Circle

Lie face up on the floor with your knees bent and your arms outstretched *(above)*. Keeping your shoulders relaxed, slowly move your arms along the floor in an arc until they are over your head. Continue the circling movement until your arms cross, then lower them over your chest. Return to the starting position.

Roll Down

Stand with your feet about 60 centimetres apart and raise your arms as if you were greeting the sky *(below, left)*. Release the muscles in your hips, unlock your knees and slowly drop forwards from the waist until your arms touch the floor. Roll back up to the start.

Single-Arm Circle

Lie on the floor with your knees bent and your arms outstretched (1). Drop your knees to the right (2) and circle your left arm over your head as you roll on to your right side (3). Continue circling your left arm downwards past your right arm (4) and, following the movement with your eyes, bring the left arm over your hip (5) and back to its original position (6).

Side-to-Side Roll

Lie on your side with your arms parallel and stretched in front of you and your legs together, extending your feet but keeping your knees bent (1). Slowly roll on to your back by opening your right arm and leg towards the right (2). Be sure to avoid arching your back. Continue rolling until you are resting on your other side (3). You can add a variation by starting out lying with your arms outstretched and your hips and legs turned to the left (4). Keep your upper body open on the floor as you open your legs and roll them to the right (5 and 6). Be sure that your knees remain slightly bent and close enough to your torso so that you avoid arching your back.

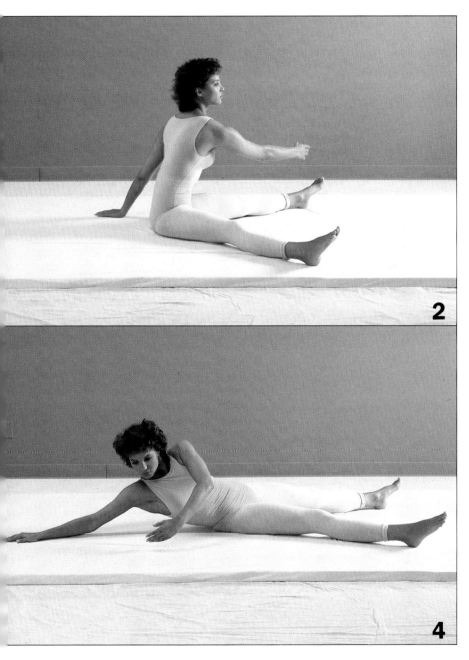

2

4

Cross Reach

Lie flat on your back with your arms and legs extended and open (1). Slide up on your left arm and reach with your right hand towards your left foot (2). Be sure not to lock your knees but keep them relaxed and slightly bent. Bend from the hips towards your foot without arching your back. Shift your support to your right arm and swing the left arm to your right foot (3). Continue the motion of your arm (4) and slide back down to the starting position, now swinging your arm over your head.

1

3

Cross Roll

Lie flat on your back with your arms and legs extended wide to form an X (1). Reach your left arm diagonally forwards to the right and sit up (2). Twist to your right and support yourself with your right hand, sliding your left arm along the floor. Then bend your right elbow and drop your chest down, untwisting your legs (3). Reach your right arm away from the floor to roll over on to your back, with your upper body open but your torso and legs still twisted to the left (4). Finally, untwist your torso, drawing your right knee across your body and up (5). Return to the starting position.

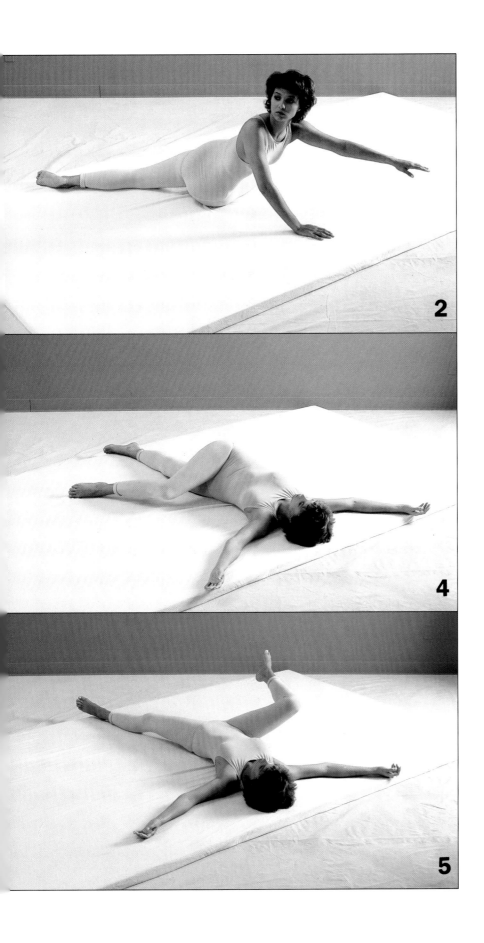

Diagonal Reach

Standing with your feet apart, reach down with your right hand towards your left foot *(right)*. Be sure that your right leg is straight and your left knee is bent. Your back should feel stretched. Then open your chest by drawing your right hand up, leading with your elbow, until your arm is fully extended.

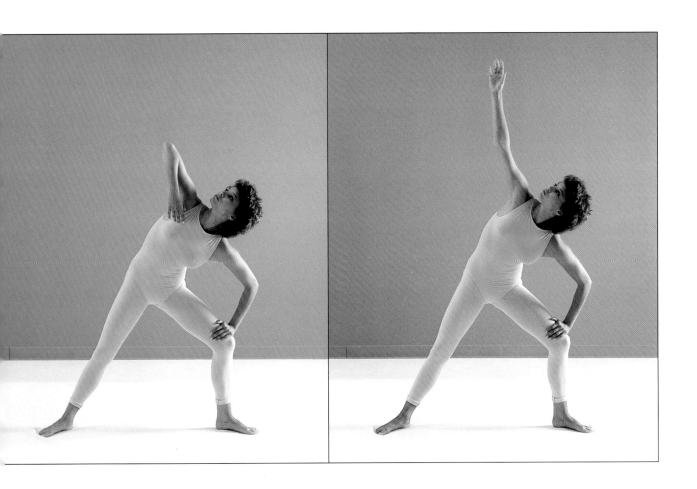

Knee-Drop Reach

Sit upright with your knees bent and your feet flat on the floor. Lean back on your hands *(left)*. Drop your knees to the left. Continue turning to your left and, supporting your body on your knees and left hand, swing your right hand up to reach over your head.

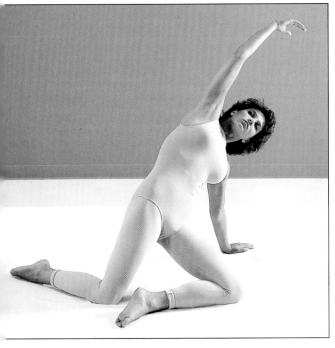

Lumbar Roll
with Lunge

Roll back on the floor, using body momentum to swing your feet towards your head (1). Do not hold that position but cross your feet and, using momentum, roll forwards (2). Separate your legs, drawing one under your body so that you can propel yourself forwards, rising up on one knee as you push forwards with your hands (3). Lifting from your hips, bring your body upwards and forwards (4). Continue to your feet in one fluid motion, swinging your arms to maintain balance (5).

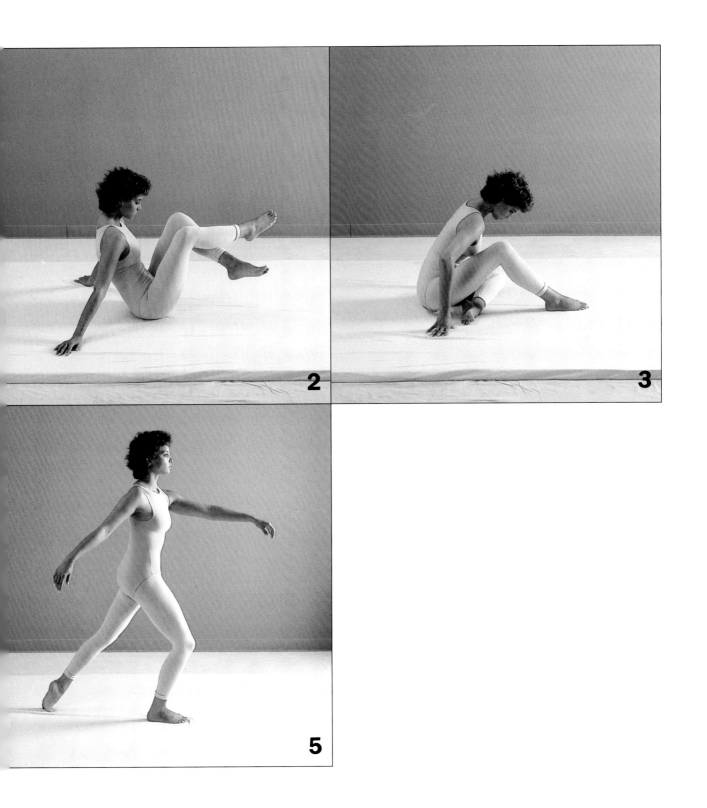

2

3

5

Twist and Sit

Stand with your arms outstretched and your feet apart (1). Keep your arms extended and twist your torso to the right (2), following with a swing of both arms. Fold your lower body (3) by bending your knees and spiralling down towards the floor (4). Catch yourself with your hands and slide down on to the floor (5), finally stretching out on your back.

1

3

Full-Body Circle

Standing with your feet apart, reach up with your left arm, stretching your left side (1). Continue your arm-reach in a circular motion (2), bending your knees slightly so that you can roll in a circle from the hips (3). Continue moving your right arm upwards (4) and follow it with your body. As you return to an erect position (5), be sure you feel the extension through the waist, not the elbow.

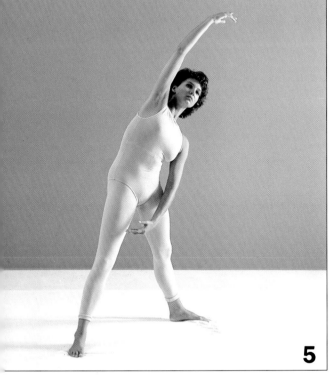

5

Salute to
the Sun

This sequence, derived from a Yoga routine, uses almost every body part. Standing with arms outstretched (1), slowly bring your hands to the floor, bending your knees slightly (2). Using your hands for support, extend one leg (3) and then the other (4) behind you, finally curling into a tucked position (5). Bring yourself out of the tuck by drawing your chest forwards (6) and extending your body forwards and up (7). Lift your hips (8), then bring one foot forwards, bringing your head up. Bring the other foot forwards, tucking your head down to your knees. Finally straighten up into a standing position, swinging your arms backwards (9).

Propulsion Sequence/1

Starting from a greet-the-sky stance (1),
swing forwards from the waist and bend
your knees (2), dropping down to a squat
(3). Dive forwards, sliding your hands
along the floor until your elbows and back
are extended (4). Bring your knees to the
floor and untuck your toes (5); curl your
body into a tucked position (6). Lift your
torso and head, drawing one knee up (7).

3

6

7

3

4

6

Propulsion
Sequence/2

You can add this sequence at the end of Propulsion Sequence/1 on pages 118-119, or you can use it as an exercise on its own. Start by sitting on your heels (1). Walk your knees forwards and come up on the balls of your feet (2). Then swing your hips backwards and sit on the floor (3). Shift your lower body forwards again, with your hips off your heels (4). Push forwards on to your knees and bring your hands beneath you to the floor, extending one leg backwards and the opposite hand forwards (5). Rise to a standing position, using your arms for balance and to achieve a smooth upward lift (6).

CHAPTER SIX

Calcium and Iron

For flexible muscles, healthy bones and optimum energy — recipes with the right amounts of these minerals

Four per cent of your body weight consists of minerals. These inorganic substances help form your skeletal structure, keep your heart beating properly and supply your muscles with oxygen. Although there are more than 60 different minerals in the human body, scientists have identified only 20 as essential. Of these, calcium and iron are two of the most important.

Calcium is critical to the flexibility and operation of your muscles. An inadequate supply can result in muscle tightness and cramps. Calcium also maintains the flexibility of the spinal column. Without enough calcium, the weight-bearing vertebrae gradually compress, reducing your range of motion. And calcium combines with phosphorus to form and preserve your bones and teeth.

If you consistently fail to get enough calcium, you increase your risk of osteoporosis — porous bones. Your bones will become weak because your body has used a great deal of its skeletal calcium to get what it needs for vital everyday functions.

A major factor behind osteoporosis is a long-term calcium deficiency that begins in the early twenties, usually because of a lack of dairy products in the diet. Some researchers suspect that a lack of exercise also contributes to the onset of the disease, which is characterized by slow, progressive bone loss. Because of hormonal differences, women suffer from osteoporosis more frequently and at an earlier age than men. But now that their average life span exceeds 70 years, osteoporosis is also increasingly evident among older men.

Two of the first signs of osteoporosis are loss of height and reduced flexibility in your back. The disease takes a long time to manifest itself and usually is only detected when a bone fracture occurs. Though it may be slowed by increasing calcium intake, osteoporosis cannot be halted entirely, possibly because the body absorbs calcium much less efficiently after the age of 60; furthermore, less of the calcium you consume goes into your bones. To minimize bone loss, people over 60 should exercise regularly and should include sources of calcium in most of their meals. But to ensure healthy bones, you should begin consuming adequate amounts of calcium when you are young. This builds up a calcium reserve that will help compensate for your body's reduced ability to absorb calcium as you get older.

The generally recommended daily amount of calcium is 500 milligrams, the equivalent of about two 25 cl (8 fl oz) glasses of milk. Unfortunately, one out of every four women gets less daily calcium than there is in one glass of milk.

The best way to get calcium is from food. Vitamin D, which is present in or added to many calcium-filled dairy products, enhances your body's calcium absorption. When you use dairy products as a source of calcium, be sure to eat and drink low-fat or skimmed-milk products to keep your fat consumption down.

On average, three quarters of our dietary calcium comes from dairy products and the rest from plant foods. Besides dairy foods, other excellent animal sources of calcium are small fish, such as sardines, that can be eaten with their soft bones intact. (The bones contain nearly all the calcium.) Tofu, molasses and leafy vegetables such as spring greens are also good sources, though not as rich as animal sources.

Weight-bearing exercises such as running, walking, hiking and aerobics increase calcium deposition in the bones of the lower body. A lack of this type of exercise slows calcium deposition, even when your dietary supply is adequate.

Your body contains much less iron than calcium: 5 grams of iron is the average as opposed to 1 to 1.5 kilograms of calcium. But iron is just as important for good health. In the red blood cells, iron plays a key role in carrying oxygen to the muscles and other organs. Without enough iron, you will lose your appetite and feel sluggish. And, as is the case with calcium, iron deficiency often starts early in life when a person's diet excludes iron-rich foods.

Men normally need about 10 milligrams of iron daily, women about

The Basic Guidelines

For a moderately active adult, Britain's National Advisory Committee on Nutrition Education recommends a diet that is low in fat, high in carbohydrates and moderate in protein. The committee's proposals for the long term suggest that no more than 30 per cent of your calories come from fat, that around 11 per cent come from protein and hence that 55 to 60 per cent come from carbohydrates. A gram of fat equals nine calories, while a gram of protein or carbohydrate equals four calories; therefore, if you eat 2,100 calories a day, you should consume approximately 70 grams of fat, 310 grams of carbohydrate and 60 grams of protein daily. If you follow a low-fat/high-carbohydrate diet, your chance of developing heart disease, cancer and other life-threatening diseases may be considerably reduced.

◆ The nutrition charts that accompany each of the low-fat/high-carbohydrate recipes in this book include the number of calories per serving, the number of grams of fat, carbohydrate and protein in a serving, and the percentage of calories derived from each of these nutrients. In addition, the charts provide the amount of calcium, iron and sodium per serving.

◆ Calcium deficiency may be associated with periodontal diseases — which attack the mouth's bones and tissues, including the gums — in both men and women, and with osteoporosis, or bone shrinking and weakening, in elderly women. The deficiency may also contribute to high blood pressure. The daily allowance for calcium recommended by the United Kingdom Department of Health and Social Security (DHSS) is 500 milligrams a day for men and women. Pregnant and lactating women are advised to consume 1,200 milligrams daily.

◆ Although one way you can reduce your fat intake is to cut your consumption of red meat, you should make sure that you get your necessary iron from other sources. The DHSS suggests a minimum of 10 milligrams of iron per day for men and 12 milligrams for women between the ages of 18 and 54.

◆ High sodium intake is associated with high blood pressure in susceptible people. Most adults should restrict sodium intake to about 2,000 milligrams a day, according to the World Health Organization. One way to keep sodium consumption in check is not to add table salt to food.

12 (because of blood loss during menstruation). The richest sources of iron are red meat, liver and egg yolks, but these also contain substantial amounts of fat and cholesterol. Good vegetarian sources are tofu, beans and iron-enriched cereals. These plant foods do not contain as much absorbable iron as animal products, but accompanying them with a small amount of meat or with foods high in vitamin C such as tomatoes or citrus fruits enhances iron absorption. Strict vegetarians, though, may well need supplemental iron during early childhood, adolescence and pregnancy. (You should take supplements only after consulting a doctor, since excessive iron intake can be toxic.)

It is a common belief that the only way to get adequate calcium and iron in your diet is by consuming relatively large quantities of milk and meat. In fact, that is not only unnecessary but unhealthy. The following recipes show how to draw on a healthy variety of sources to provide these two essential minerals.

Breakfast

HERBED MELON WITH YOGURT SAUCE

Studies of football players, cross-country runners and other athletes show that weight-bearing exercise strengthens the bones of the lower body. This breakfast of melon and yogurt provides plenty of calcium, another way to help keep your bones strong.

2 tablespoons honey
1½ tablespoons lemon juice
4 tablespoons finely chopped
   fresh basil
2 tablespoons finely chopped
   fresh mint

½ teaspoon coarsely ground black
   pepper
1 medium-sized cantaloupe melon
25 cl (8 fl oz) plain low-fat yogurt

CALORIES	240
77% Carbohydrate	50 g
14% Protein	9 g
9% Fat	3 g
CALCIUM	290 mg
IRON	2 mg
SODIUM	106 mg

Combine 1 tablespoon of the honey, the lemon juice, 1½ tablespoons of the basil, ½ tablespoon of the mint and ¼ teaspoon of the pepper in a large bowl. Cut the melon into 4 cm (1½ inch) cubes, add it to the bowl and toss to coat. Combine the yogurt, remaining honey, herbs and pepper in a small bowl and stir well. Let the sauce stand for 15 minutes to allow the flavours to blend. Divide the melon and sauce between two shallow bowls.   Makes 2 servings

CORIANDER AND CURRANT SCONES

You can add calcium to your diet in cooked foods such as these scones. The buttermilk they contain is an excellent low-fat calcium source.

125 g (4 oz) wholemeal flour
150 g (5 oz) plain flour
1 tablespoon baking powder
2½ teaspoons ground coriander
½ teaspoon salt
½ teaspoon sugar

45 g (1½ oz) unsalted butter,
   well chilled
125 g (4 oz) currants or raisins
1 tablespoon grated orange rind
17.5 cl (6 fl oz) buttermilk

CALORIES per scone	400
70% Carbohydrate	71 g
8% Protein	8 g
22% Fat	10 g
CALCIUM	255 mg
IRON	3 mg
SODIUM	733 mg

Combine the dry ingredients in a medium-sized bowl. With two knives, cut in the butter until the mixture resembles breadcrumbs. Scatter in the currants and orange rind, then stir in the buttermilk with a fork until just combined. Turn the dough out on to a floured board and knead it with floured hands three or four times. Lightly grease a baking sheet. Divide the dough into four equal portions and shape each into a ball. Flatten the balls of dough with the palm of the hand. Place the balls of dough on the baking sheet. With a sharp knife cut a deep cross in the top of each, then refrigerate for 15 minutes. Meanwhile, preheat the oven to 220°C (425°F or Mark 7). Bake the scones for about 15 minutes, or until golden-brown.   Makes 4 scones

Variation: for Shortcake Scones, omit the wholemeal flour and use 300 g (10 oz) of plain flour; omit the coriander, orange rind and currants. Roll the dough out 3 cm (1¼ inches) thick on a floured board and cut with an 8.5 cm (3½ inch) round or heart-shaped biscuit cutter. Bake as directed above. Use the scones for Fig-Berry Shortcakes (see page 137) and other desserts.

KASHA WITH YOGURT AND BLUEBERRIES

Cooking the kasha in semi-skimmed milk (a complete protein) helps your body to make full use of the incomplete protein in the grain.

CALORIES	140
73% Carbohydrate	26 g
20% Protein	7 g
7% Fat	1 g
CALCIUM	225 mg
IRON	1 mg
SODIUM	120 mg

50 cl (16 fl oz) semi-skimmed milk
100 g (3½ oz) coarse kasha
   (toasted buckwheat groats)
½ teaspoon ground cinnamon
Dash of salt

12.5 cl (4 fl oz) plain low-fat
   yogurt
4 teaspoons brown sugar
150 g (5 oz) fresh blueberries, or
   frozen blueberries, thawed

In a small saucepan over medium-high heat, bring the milk to the boil. Gradually stir in the kasha, then the cinnamon and salt. Reduce the heat to low and cook, stirring occasionally, for about 10 minutues, or until the milk is absorbed. Spoon the kasha into four bowls and top each serving with 2 tablespoons of yogurt, a teaspoon of sugar and a quarter of the blueberries.　Makes 4 servings

Coriander and Currant Scones

SWEET POTATO SLICES WITH SMOKED PORK LOIN

Iron-rich molasses is the only sweetener that provides significant nutrients. According to many sports doctors, you can improve your iron absorption by not drinking coffee or tea (which inhibit iron uptake) with your meals.

2 tablespoons maple syrup
1 tablespoon dark molasses
4 tablespoons cornmeal
¾ teaspoon sugar
⅛ teaspoon salt

1 large orange-fleshed sweet
   potato (about 250g/8 oz), boiled
   and peeled
15 g (½ oz) unsalted butter
2 thin slices smoked pork loin

In a small bowl, stir together the maple syrup and molasses. Combine the cornmeal, sugar and salt in a shallow dish. Slice the potato into rounds 5 mm (¼ inch) thick and dredge in the cornmeal mixture until completely coated. Melt half of the butter in a large, heavy non-stick frying pan over medium-high heat. Place a single layer of potato slices in the pan and cook for about 5 minutes, or until the undersides are lightly browned. Turn the potatoes, add the remaining butter to the pan and cook for another 5 minutes, or until lightly browned. Transfer the potatoes to a plate and wipe the pan with paper towels. Add the pork to the pan and sear it over medium-high heat for about 1 minute on each side, or until browned. Transfer the pork to the plate with the potatoes and serve with the maple-molasses syrup.   Makes 1 serving.

CALORIES	555
70% Carbohydrate	99 g
7% Protein	10 g
23% Fat	14 g
CALCIUM	230 mg
IRON	6 mg
SODIUM	726 mg

Sweet Potato Slices with Smoked Pork Loin

Chilled Mango Soup

Lunch

CHILLED MANGO SOUP

A milk-based soup like this one will add extra calcium to a meal.

1 large ripe mango (about 500 g/
   1 lb)
50 cl (16 fl oz) buttermilk
4 tablespoons dried skimmed milk
4 tablespoons lime juice
25 cl (8 fl oz) soda water

½ cucumber, seeded and finely
   diced
1 small fresh hot red chili
   pepper, chopped
4 teaspoons finely chopped fresh
   coriander, basil or mint

Halve and stone the mango and scoop the flesh into the goblet of a blender. Add the buttermilk, dried milk and lime juice, and purée until smooth. (This mixture can be made in advance and refrigerated until serving time.) Just before serving, stir in the soda water and divide the soup among four bowls. Divide the cucumber equally among the bowls and sprinkle each serving with the chili pepper and herbs.
Makes 4 servings

CALORIES	135
72% Carbohydrate	26 g
19% Protein	7 g
9% Fat	1 g
CALCIUM	220 mg
IRON	Trace
SODIUM	156 mg

Pasta with Goat Cheese and Onions

PASTA WITH GOAT CHEESE AND ONIONS

Fortified skimmed milk contains vitamin D, a nutrient that aids calcium absorption. Although your skin produces vitamin D when exposed to sunlight, studies made in the United States show that the skin's ability to manufacture vitamin D decreases with age.

175 g (6 oz) mild French goat cheese	**Black pepper**
12.5 cl (4 fl oz) skimmed milk	**4 tablespoons finely chopped fresh herbs in any combination,**
1 medium-sized red onion	**such as basil, chives, flat-leaf**
½ teaspoon olive oil	**parsley, coriander, thyme or**
250 g (8 oz) capelletti or small shell pasta	**rosemary**
	1½ teaspoons grated Parmesan

CALORIES	470
54% Carbohydrate	63 g
18% Protein	21 g
28% Fat	15 g
CALCIUM	334 mg
IRON	3 mg
SODIUM	580 mg

Bring enough water to the boil in the bottom of a double boiler so that the boiling water will just touch the top pan. When the water boils, place the goat cheese in the top pan and heat, stirring with a whisk, until the cheese is completely melted. Whisk in the skimmed milk, cover the pan and set aside.

Bring a large pan of water to the boil. Preheat the grill and position the rack 5 cm (2 inches) from the heat. Slice the onion into wedges 3 mm (⅛ inch) thick; do not separate the layers. Place a non-stick baking sheet under the grill for 1 minute, or until hot. Arrange the onion wedges in a single layer on the sheet and brush the tops and sides of the slices lightly with the oil. Grill the onions for about 5 minutes, or until they are soft and slightly charred.

Cook the pasta in the boiling water until *al dente*, drain well and return to the pan. Add the cheese mixture, some black pepper and half the fresh herbs and toss well. Divide the pasta among three dinner plates and top with equal amounts of charred onions and Parmesan. Sprinkle with the remaining herbs and serve immediately. Makes 3 servings

VEGETABLE-CHEESE BURRITOS

Spinach and other dark leafy greens are high in iron, fibre, potassium, vitamin A and vitamin C.

CALORIES	390
38% Carbohydrate	39 g
13% Protein	12 g
49% Fat	21 g
CALCIUM	285 mg
IRON	2 mg
SODIUM	537 mg

125 g (4 oz) rocket, watercress or spinach leaves, coarsely chopped
1 large tomato, cored and cut into 2.5 cm (1 inch) pieces
90 g (3 oz) feta cheese, crumbled
1 tablespoon finely chopped red onion

1 sweet red pepper, roasted, peeled and finely diced
1 garlic clove, crushed
1 tablespoon red wine vinegar, preferably balsamic
1½ teaspoons dried oregano
Six 20 cm (8 inch) flour tortillas (recipe follows)

Combine the chopped greens, tomato, feta, onion, red pepper, garlic and vinegar in a large bowl. Heat a large frying pan over high heat. Sprinkle ¼ teaspoon of the oregano over the surface of the pan. When the oregano is just smoking, add one tortilla and heat for about 30 seconds. Remove the tortilla from the pan and place one sixth of the vegetable mixture in the centre. Fold the bottom third of the tortilla over the filling, then roll the sides together loosely. Repeat with the remaining tortillas and filling, and serve. Makes 3 servings

FLOUR TORTILLAS

150 g (6 oz) plain flour   **45 g (1½ oz) white vegetable fat**
⅓ teaspoon salt

Mix the flour with the salt and rub in the fat. Gradually add 4½ tablespoons of warm water and knead the dough for 3 minutes. Put the dough in a bowl, cover it with plastic film and leave it to rest at room temperature for 15 minutes. Divide the dough into six equal pieces and roll each piece out on a floured board to make a 20 cm (8 inch) circle.

Cook each tortilla in a lightly greased non-stick frying pan or crepe pan until bubbles form and the surface is lightly speckled — about 30 seconds. Using a wooden spoon or spatula, flatten the bubbles, then turn the tortilla over and cook it for 30 seconds on the other side. Makes six 20 cm (8 inch) flour tortillas

CALORIES per tortilla	150
46% Carbohydrate	18 g
8% Protein	3 g
46% Fat	8 g
CALCIUM	35 mg
IRON	Trace
SODIUM	65 mg

FRITTATA WITH GREENS AND TOFU

This quick lunch or dinner dish gets its iron boost from tofu and greens, and is an excellent source of protein as well as calcium.

500 g (1 lb) trimmed mustard
   or spring greens, coarsely
   chopped
1½ teaspoons olive oil
90 g (3 oz) shallots, coarsely
   chopped
6 garlic cloves, crushed
2 whole anchovies, with bones,
   rinsed, dried and finely chopped

¼ teaspoon hot red pepper flakes
1 teaspoon dried thyme
175 g (6 oz) firm tofu, cut into
   5 mm (¼ inch) cubes
3 large eggs
3 tablespoons skimmed milk
¼ teaspoon salt
45 g (1½ oz) low-fat mozzarella,
   cut into thin strips

Place the greens in a large non-stick frying pan with 12.5 cl (4 fl oz) of water, cover and cook over medium-low heat for about 20 minutes, or until tender. Uncover the pan and cook until the moisture evaporates. Transfer the greens to a large bowl; set aside.

Heat the oil in a large non-stick frying pan over medium heat. Add the shallots, garlic, anchovies, red pepper flakes and thyme, and cook for about 10 minutes, or until the shallots and garlic are softened. Add the greens and tofu to the pan, toss to coat well and distribute the mixture evenly in the pan.

In a medium-sized bowl, beat together the eggs, milk and salt and pour the mixture into the pan, pressing the egg mixture evenly into the greens and tofu with a wooden spoon. Cook, covered, over medium heat for 3 to 4 minutes, or until the eggs are set. Lay the mozzarella strips on top of the frittata, reduce the heat to low, cover and cook for about 1 minute, or just until the cheese melts. Serve hot or warm.   Makes 4 servings

CALORIES	200
29% Carbohydrate	16 g
29% Protein	16 g
42% Fat	10 g
CALCIUM	308 mg
IRON	4 mg
SODIUM	295 mg

HEARTY SQUASH SOUP

The acorn squash used in this thick, rich soup is a good source of iron and provides a substantial amount of vitamin A and protein.

2 acorn squashes (750 g/1½ lb
   each)
4 tablespoons low-sodium
   chicken stock
4 large shallots, finely chopped
1 teaspoon olive oil
2 tablespoons dry white wine
12.5 cl (4 fl oz) evaporated milk
¾ teaspoon black pepper

¼ teaspoon salt
Four 5 mm (¼ inch) slices
   wholemeal bread
75 g (2½ oz) low-fat mozzarella,
   grated
60 g (2 oz) Gruyère cheese, grated
2 tablespoons finely chopped
   fresh basil

Preheat the oven to 200°C (400°F or Mark 6). Cut off a 4 cm (1½ inch) "lid" from the stem end of each squash. Cut a thin slice off the bottom of each squash, then scoop out and discard the seeds and stringy membranes. Place the squashes upright and the lids cut side up on a foil-lined baking sheet. Place 2 tablespoons of the stock in each squash and cover loosely with foil. Bake for 40 minutes, or until the squashes are just tender but still hold their shape.

CALORIES	640
57% Carbohydrate	95 g
19% Protein	33 g
24% Fat	18 g
CALCIUM	985 mg
IRON	6 mg
SODIUM	878 mg

Meanwhile, in a small saucepan over medium heat sauté the shallots in the oil until they just begin to brown. Add the wine and cook, stirring, until it evaporates. Remove the pan from the heat. When the squashes are cooked, carefully scoop out the flesh with a teaspoon, leaving a 1 cm (½ inch) shell and being careful not to pierce the skin. Add the scooped-out flesh, the milk, pepper and salt to the shallots and cook over medium heat until hot, mashing the squash with a wooden spoon. Spoon one sixth of the mixture into each hollowed-out squash and top with some bread. Sprinkle with one sixth of the cheese and top with another sixth of the squash mixture. Repeat the layers of bread, squash and cheese until the squashes are filled, finishing with a layer of cheese. Return the lids and squashes to the oven and bake for 10 minutes, or until the cheese has melted. Sprinkle each serving with basil, cover the squashes with the lids and serve. Makes 2 servings

SARDINE CAKES WITH TARRAGON-MUSTARD SAUCE

Always eat sardines with the bones, which are the source of calcium.

2 leeks	**1 large egg**
1 tablespoon olive oil	**¼ teaspoon dried thyme**
150 g (5 oz) brine-packed sardines, drained	**⅛ teaspoon black pepper**
	1 teaspoon grated lemon rind
2 medium-sized potatoes (about 500 g/1 lb), boiled in their skins, peeled and mashed	**¼ teaspoon anchovy paste**
	Tarragon-Mustard Sauce (recipe follows)

Trim the leeks, discarding the green leaves. Split and carefully wash the leeks and slice them thinly. Heat the oil in a small frying pan over medium-high heat, add the leeks and cook for about 6 minutes, or until softened. Add 1 tablespoon of water to prevent sticking, if necessary. Set aside to cool. With a fork, mash the sardines in a large bowl. Add the leeks, potatoes, egg, thyme, black pepper, lemon rind and anchovy paste, and stir to combine. Heat a large non-stick frying pan over medium-high heat. Form the sardine mixture into 12 equally sized patties and cook for about 2 minutes on each side, or until browned. Serve with Tarragon-Mustard sauce. Makes 6 servings

CALORIES without sauce	165
41% Carbohydrate	17 g
17% Protein	7 g
42% Fat	8 g
CALCIUM	99 mg
IRON	1 mg
SODIUM	255 mg

TARRAGON-MUSTARD SAUCE

1 teaspoon dry mustard	**2 teaspoons finely chopped parsley**
4 tablespoons juice from dill-pickled cucumber	**4 tablespoons finely chopped dill-pickled cucumber**
2 teaspoons dried tarragon	
12.5 cl (4 fl oz) Greek yogurt	**½ teaspoon crushed garlic**
	⅛ teaspoon sugar
4 teaspoons finely chopped shallot	

In a medium-sized bowl dissolve the mustard in the pickle juice. Add the tarragon and set aside for 5 minutes. Add the yogurt, shallot, parsley, pickled cucumber, garlic and sugar, and stir to combine. Makes 25 cl (8 fl oz)

CALORIES per tablespoon	15
25% Carbohydrate	1 g
8% Protein	0.4 g
67% Fat	1 g
CALCIUM	5 mg
IRON	Trace
SODIUM	166 mg

Dinner

LIVER AND FIGS EN BROCHETTE

Although liver is an outstanding source of iron, protein and B vitamins, it also contains a fair amount of saturated fat and cholesterol. You should not eat it more than twice a week.

CALORIES	505
52% Carbohydrate	70 g
23% Protein	29 g
25% Fat	14 g
CALCIUM	218 mg
IRON	10 mg
SODIUM	600 mg

2 red onions (about 600 g/1¼ lb)
1 tablespoon dry sherry
2⅔ tablespoons olive oil
1 teaspoon dried thyme, crushed
½ teaspoon dried sage, crumbled
½ teaspoon coarsely ground black pepper
4 garlic cloves, crushed

⅜ teaspoon salt
12 bay leaves
350 g (12 oz) calf's liver, cut into sixteen 2.5 cm (1 inch) cubes
6 fresh figs, halved
1 baguette (slender loaf of French bread)

Leaving the root end intact, cut each onion lengthwise into six to eight 2.5 cm (1 inch) wide wedges. In a medium-sized bowl, combine the sherry, 1 tablespoon of the olive oil, the thyme, sage, pepper, garlic and ¼ teaspoon of the salt. Add the onions, bay leaves and liver and toss to coat with the marinade. Cover and marinate in the refrigerator for 3 to 4 hours or overnight.

Preheat the grill and position the rack 10 cm (4 inches) from the heat. Alternately thread 4 liver cubes, 3 bay leaves and 3 fig halves on to each of four 20 to 25 cm (8 to 10 inch) skewers. Lay the onion wedges on a baking sheet,

Liver and Figs en Brochette

brush them with 1 teaspoon of the oil and sprinkle them with the remaining salt. Cut the baguette diagonally into twelve 1 cm (½ inch) slices and brush the slices with the remaining oil; set aside. Grill the onions, turning them half way through cooking, for about 7 minutes, or until they are soft. Divide the onions among four plates. Place the bread slices on a baking sheet and grill them for about 1½ minutes, or until lightly browned on top. Transfer the bread to the plates. Place the brochettes on a grill pan and grill for 4 to 5 minutes, until the liver is browned; turn the brochettes and grill for a further 4 to 5 minutes. Do not worry if the bay leaves smoke a bit. Transfer the skewers to the plates and serve.

Makes 4 servings

LINGUINE WITH FIGS AND WALNUTS

This dish would be good to include in a recovery meal following an endurance event. The cheese is an excellent source of protein and calcium, and the figs supply potassium, an important mineral lost in perspiration.

CALORIES	695
62% Carbohydrate	109g
11% Protein	21g
27% Fat	22 g
CALCIUM	374 mg
IRON	6 mg
SODIUM	571 mg

2 tablespoons olive oil, preferably extra-virgin
7 garlic cloves, peeled and thinly sliced
2 anchovy fillets, rinsed, dried and finely chopped
3 leeks, white part only, thinly sliced
10 dried figs, cut into 1 cm x 3 mm (½ x ⅛ inch) pieces
1 tablespoon dry white wine
5 tablespoons low-sodium chicken stock
30 g (1 oz) shelled walnuts, coarsely chopped
4 tablespoons finely chopped flat-leaf parsley
250 g (8 oz) linguine or spaghetti
¼ teaspoon salt
Black pepper
45 g (1½ oz) Parmesan, grated

Bring a large saucepan of water to the boil. Meanwhile, for the sauce, heat 1 tablespoon of the oil in a medium-sized non-stick frying pan over medium heat. Add the garlic and sauté for about 5 minutes, or until the garlic just begins to brown. Stir in the anchovy fillets, then add the leeks and figs. Cover the pan, reduce the heat slightly and cook for about 8 minutes, or until the leeks are tender. Stir in the wine and cook for 45 seconds. Stir in the chicken stock, walnuts and half of the parsley and cook for another minute. Remove the pan from the heat, cover to keep warm and set aside.

Cook the linguine in the boiling water until *al dente*, drain and return to the saucepan. Add the remaining olive oil and parsley, the salt and some pepper, and toss. Divide the linguine between two bowls and spoon an equal amount of sauce and Parmesan over each. Serve immediately.   Makes 2 servings

SEAFOOD AND BROCCOLI SALAD WITH BLACK BEAN DRESSING

Scallops are high in protein and iron, and also lower in cholesterol than most shellfish. Steaming vegetables rather than boiling them preserves the maximum amount of nutrients.

1 tablespoon safflower oil
2 tablespoons chopped fresh
   ginger root
1½ tablespoons chopped garlic
4 tablespoons chopped spring
   onions
¼ teaspoon hot red pepper flakes
1 tablespoon Chinese salted
   black beans, rinsed
2 teaspoons low-sodium soy
   sauce or shoyu

2 teaspoons Japanese rice-wine
   vinegar
350 g (12 oz) broccoli, cut into
   2.5 cm (1 inch) florets, stems
   peeled and cut into 1 cm (½ inch)
   pieces
125 g (4 oz) medium-sized raw
   prawns in shell
125 g (4 oz) shelled scallops
Small firm pear, such as a
   Conference

For the dressing, heat the oil in a large frying pan over medium-high heat. Add the ginger, garlic, spring onions, pepper flakes and black beans, and cook for 5 to 6 minutes, or until the garlic is golden. Add the soy sauce, vinegar and 1 tablespoon of water, and cook for another 30 seconds. Transfer the mixture to a medium-sized bowl and set aside.

Bring 2.5 cm (1 inch) of water to the boil in a covered saucepan large enough to hold a vegetable steamer. When the water boils, place the broccoli and prawns in the steamer, cover, and cook for about 4 minutes, or until the broccoli is bright green and the prawns are pink and almost cooked. Add the scallops and steam for another minute. Transfer the broccoli and scallops to the bowl of dressing. Peel the prawns, add to the broccoli and scallops, and toss well. Divide the salad between two plates, reserving some of the dressing. Halve, core and peel the pear and cut it into 5 mm (¼ inch) dice. Toss the diced pear with the reserved dressing and place in the centre of each serving of salad.

Makes 2 servings

CALORIES	265
38% Carbohydrate	27 g
36% Protein	25 g
26% Fat	8 g
CALCIUM	162 mg
IRON	4 mg
SODIUM	462 mg

Note: Chinese salted black beans (sometimes called fermented black beans) are soya beans that have been cooked, seasoned and then aged for several months. They are used in small amounts for flavouring. Salted black beans are sold in cans or plastic bags in Chinese food shops and will keep indefinitely in a tightly closed jar at room temperature. Japanese rice-wine vinegar is mild and slightly sweet. Substitute mild cider vinegar or white distilled vinegar if rice-wine vinegar is unavailable.

Fig-Berry Shortcakes

Desserts

FIG-BERRY SHORTCAKES

Besides containing iron and calcium, figs are also extremely high in fibre. Be sure to drink plenty of fluids with them to aid digestion.

10 dried figs
½ vanilla pod, split, seeds
scraped out and reserved
250 g (8 oz) each strawberries and
raspberries
2 tablespoons honey

4 Shortcake Scones (see
Coriander and Currant Scones
recipe, page 126)
12.5 cl (4 fl oz) Honey Cream
(recipe follows)

CALORIES	570
71% Carbohydrate	105 g
10% Protein	15 g
19% Fat	13 g
CALCIUM	336 mg
IRON	4 mg
SODIUM	769 mg

For the fig-berry sauce, place the figs and the vanilla pod halves and seeds in a 1 litre (2 pint) saucepan, add water to cover and bring to the boil. Reduce the heat and simmer for about 10 minutes, or until the figs are tender. Meanwhile, wash the berries and hull and slice the strawberries. Combine half each of the raspberries and strawberries with the honey in a food processor, and purée. Strain the purée into a medium-sized bowl and set aside. When the figs are cooked, drain them and, when cool enough to handle, quarter them and cut into thin slices. Reserving a few berries for garnish, stir the remaining berries and the figs into the purée. Chill the mixture until ready to serve.

To serve, split the scones in half. Spoon a quarter of the fig-berry sauce on to the bottom of each scone, then top with 2 tablespoons of Honey Cream. Cover with the scone tops and garnish with whole berries if desired.   Makes 4 servings

HONEY CREAM

CALORIES per tablespoon	20
26% Carbohydrate	1 g
37% Protein	2 g
37% Fat	1 g
CALCIUM	9 mg
IRON	Trace
SODIUM	59 mg

Use this low-fat alternative to whipped cream as a topping on fresh or cooked fruit to create desserts that are rich in calcium yet lower in fat. It can also replace butter and syrup on griddle cakes or waffles.

250 (8 oz) quark (0% fat)
2 teaspoons honey

5 tablespoons Greek yogurt

Put the quark in a small bowl and fold in the honey and yogurt. Cover the bowl and refrigerate the mixture until ready to use. Honey Cream will keep for a week refrigerated in a covered container. Makes 25 cl (8 fl oz)

GINGER SOUFFLÉS

This dish supplies complete protein as well as healthy amounts of vitamins and minerals. The sweet potatoes provide protein, vitamin A and potassium as well as vitamin C, which aids the body's absorption of the iron from the molasses. The egg whites add extra protein without the cholesterol which is present in egg yolks. Dried skimmed milk is packed with protein and calcium but contains little fat.

2 medium-sized orange-fleshed sweet potatoes (about 350 g/ 12 oz total weight), boiled, peeled and cut into chunks
4 tablespoons dried skimmed milk
2 tablespoons evaporated milk
45 g (1½ oz) crystallized ginger, chopped
2 tablespoons grated fresh ginger root

4 teaspoons molasses
1 tablespoon honey
½ teaspoon pure vanilla extract
2 eggs, separated, plus 4 egg whites
⅛ teaspoon cream of tartar
⅛ teaspoon salt
3 tablespoons sugar

CALORIES	280
69% Carbohydrate	52 g
18% Protein	13 g
13% Fat	4 g
CALCIUM	260 mg
IRON	4 mg
SODIUM	210 mg

Preheat the oven to 220°C (425°F or Mark 7). Grease four 35 cl (12 fl oz) individual soufflé or baking dishes. Place the dishes on a baking sheet and set aside. Purée the sweet potatoes in a food processor until perfectly smooth, then transfer the purée to a medium-sized bowl. Whisk in the dried milk, evaporated milk, crystallized and fresh ginger, molasses, honey, vanilla and the 2 egg yolks. In another medium-sized bowl, using an electric mixer beat the 6 egg whites, the cream of tartar and the salt until soft peaks form. While continuing to beat, sprinkle in the sugar 1 tablespoon at a time and beat until stiff peaks form. Using a rubber spatula, fold one third of the whites into the sweet potato mixture, then gently fold in the remaining whites until incorporated, being careful not to deflate the mixture.

Divide the mixture among the prepared soufflé dishes, mounding slightly in the centres. Place the baking sheet with the soufflés in the oven and immediately reduce the temperature to 190°C (375°F or Mark 5). Bake the soufflés for 15 to 17 minutes, or until they are puffed and browned. Serve immediately. Makes 4 servings

FRESH FRUIT WITH CUSTARD

Iron from plant sources such as raspberries is not as well absorbed by the body as the iron in animal foods. But accompanying such iron sources with foods rich in vitamin C (such as the strawberries in this recipe) will enhance the amount of iron your body absorbs.

50 cl (16 fl oz) evaporated milk
4 tablespoons honey
Three 2.5 x 7.5 cm (1 x 3 inch)
   strips orange peel
1½ teaspoons fennel seeds
1 vanilla pod, split, seeds
   scraped out and reserved
3 egg yolks

250 g (8 oz) each strawberries and
   raspberries, or 500 g (1 lb)
   of either
2 nectarines or peaches,
   thinly sliced
4 amaretti (Italian almond
   biscuits), coarsely crushed

For the custard, bring enough water to the boil in the bottom of a double boiler so that the boiling water will just touch the top pan. In the top pan combine the milk, honey, orange peel, fennel seeds and vanilla pod halves and seeds. Cook, covered, over the boiling water for 15 minutes. Whisk in the egg yolks and cook, uncovered, stirring occasionally, for about 15 minutes, or until the mixture coats the back of a wooden spoon. Reduce the heat and keep the custard warm until ready to serve.

Just before serving, wash and dry the berries and hull and slice the strawberries, if using. Mound half of the berries on four dessert plates and lay the nectarine slices pinwheel-fashion on top. Arrange the remaining berries decoratively on the plate. Strain the warm custard into a measuring jug; discard the vanilla pod and seeds and the orange peel. Pour 4 tablespoons of custard over each serving, then sprinkle the fruit and custard with the crushed amaretti.

Makes 4 servings

Note: amaretti are Italian almond macaroons made without egg yolks or shortening. They are sold in delicatessens and many supermarkets. If amaretti are unavailable, substitute other plain biscuits.

CALORIES	355
42% Carbohydrate	39 g
16% Protein	14 g
42% Fat	17 g
CALCIUM	390 mg
IRON	3 mg
SODIUM	236 mg

Snacks and Beverages

ANTIPASTO SNACK

This mixture of pickled fruits and vegetables, a variation on an Italian condiment, makes a delicious snack or appetizer. The okra and dried fruits supply calcium, potassium and fibre, and the apricots, like most deep-yellow fruits and vegetables, are also rich in vitamin A.

CALORIES	400
68% Carbohydrate	71 g
13% Protein	14 g
19% Fat	9 g
CALCIUM	346 mg
IRON	4 mg
SODIUM	488 mg

750 g (1½ lb) fresh okra
350 g (12 oz) stoned prunes (about 40)
500 g (1 lb) onions, peeled and thinly sliced
125 g (4 oz) dried apricots (about 16)
1 sprig fresh thyme
1 medium-sized fresh or dried hot red chili pepper

4 garlic cloves, peeled
1 litre (1 ¾ pints) white wine vinegar
2 tablespoons coriander seeds
2 tablespoons sugar
¼ teaspoon coarse salt
4 bay leaves
250 g (8 oz) provolone cheese
16 breadsticks

Antipasto Snack

Wash and trim the okra and pack the pods vertically into a 3 litre (5 pint) preserving jar. Toss the prunes with the onion slices and place the mixture on top of the okra. Place the apricots on top of the prunes and onions and tuck the thyme sprig, chili pepper and garlic cloves down into the jar. In a non-reactive saucepan combine 75 cl (1¼ pints) of water with the vinegar, coriander seeds, sugar, salt and bay leaves, and bring to a rolling boil. Pour the boiling liquid into the jar, filling it to the top. Let cool, then close the jar tightly and refrigerate for two to three days to allow the flavours to develop. Accompany each serving with 30 g (1 oz) of provolone and two breadsticks.   Makes 8 servings

CRANBERRY-WALNUT COMPOTE

Spread this compote on slices of wholemeal bread, or stir it into plain low-fat yogurt, to enrich with calcium, protein, iron and fibre. It can also be served as a relish with poultry.

500 g (1 lb) fresh or frozen cranberries	**175 g (6 oz) shelled walnuts, coarsely chopped**
3 navel oranges, skins left on, quartered and thinly sliced	**4 tablespoons lime or lemon juice, preferably freshly squeezed**
250 g (8 oz) honey	
175 g (6 oz) raisins	

In a heavy non-reactive 3 litre (5 pint) saucepan, combine 400 g (14 oz) of the cranberries, the oranges, honey and 35 cl (12 fl oz) of hot water, and bring to the boil over medium-high heat. Reduce the heat to medium and cook, stirring occasionally, for about 15 minutes, or until the mixture has thickened and the cranberries are soft. Stir in the raisins and remaining cranberries and cook for another 4 minutes, or until the raisins are plump. Remove the pan from the heat and stir in the walnuts and juice. Transfer the compote to a glass or ceramic bowl, crock or jar, cover and chill before serving.   Makes 2 litres (3½ pints)

CALORIES per 8 cl (3 fl oz)	115
68% Carbohydrate	22 g
5% Protein	2 g
27% Fat	4 g
CALCIUM	26 mg
IRON	5 mg
SODIUM	3 mg

ORANGE REFRESHER

This drink provides just as much calcium as a milk shake, but it has less fat and refined sugar, and more protein, vitamin C and potassium.

17.5 cl (6 fl oz) orange juice, preferably freshly squeezed	**Fresh mint sprig for garnish (optional)**
3½ tablespoons dried skimmed milk	**Fresh orange slices for garnish (optional)**
3 ice cubes	

Place the orange juice, dried milk and ice cubes in a blender and blend until frothy. Pour the drink into a tall glass and garnish with a mint sprig and orange slices if desired.   Makes 1 serving

CALORIES	135
78% Carbohydrate	27 g
19% Protein	7 g
3% Fat	0.5 g
CALCIUM	204 mg
IRON	Trace
SODIUM	84 mg

PROP CREDITS

Page 127, tablecloth: Vantona, Saville Row, London W1; cutlery:
Oneida; plate: Inshop, 18 New Cavendish Street, London W1;
page 134, tablecloth: Next Interiors.

ACKNOWLEDGEMENTS

The Editors wish to thank Kate Cann and Norma MacMillan.

PHOTOGRAPHY CREDIT

All photographs by Steven Mays, Rebus, Inc., except photographs
pages 127, 129 and 134: Chris Knaggs.

ILLUSTRATION CREDITS

All illustrations by David Flaherty except illustrations pages 20-21:
Stuart Bragg.

INDEX